A Patient's View of Nurses and Doctors

John F. Sueta

Dedication

I owe a large debt of gratitude to the following people. Every ward, in every hospital, needs such exceptional people who go beyond the normal call of duty and give their best.

Nurses: Maryann Latorre, RN, Gisela Rosa, RN, Shirley Redden, RN, Theresa Palacio, RN, Violetta Delamerced, RN, Gary Abrams, RN, Linda Robinson, RN, Anne Holkias, RN, Venida Charuratna, RN, Elizabeth Hunt, RN, Linda Pearce, RN, Desdemona Agard, RN, and Florette E. Cramer, RN.

Doctors: I would be remiss if I did not thank a few outstanding doctors who were critically important to my recovery: Howard Singer, MD, Elliot Abemayor, MD, Michael Sochat, MD, Natacha Sochat, MD, Masahiro Suguwara, MD, and __ Finch, MD.

Nursing Aides: Pat Norby, CNA, and P.Castle, CNA. Nursing aides deserve special recognition. They are a hardworking and devoted group of people who do much of the unpleasant duties of patient care and receive very little recognition, respect, and monetary reward. They are a very important part of nursing.

Physical Therapists: Rick Phillips, Douglas Hudgens, Joe Glenn, and Mary __.

Supporting friends: Hugh and Barbara Whelpton, George and Flo Kallas, David Lee Williams, Bill Dickson, Robert Sax, Virginia Karnosky, Tom Rauscher, Althea John, and Charlene Williams.

And lastly, I want to express my appreciation to Wadsworth Veterans Hospital in West Los Angeles for their excellent care.

Introduction

The following story is about human beings joined together in one of the most complex human interactions possible, that intense relationship that occurs between hospital patients and medical personnel.

The story of my fight against a paralyzing illness is merely the vehicle for telling the more important underlying story of the compassion of medical personnel and the great work they do under incredibly difficult conditions.

The journey is a path that wends its way through dozens of medical and interpersonal situations. On the path, the attitudes, behaviors, and skills of medical people are described from a patient's point of view. Conversely, my own feelings and behavior, both good and bad, are revealed as I interact with my caregivers.

Many important issues are covered along the way. They are serious topics, but I tried to explain them simply, with a light-hearted touch.

Medical issues:

An explanation of stress, its causes, effects, and ways to cope with it.

An update of what's being done in paralysis research and treatment.

Common hospital errors and what can be done about them.

The method of weaning a patient off a ventilator.

Nursing issues:

Examples of good and bad nursing.

The benefits of having a primary nurse rather than team nursing.

The value of tough love.

How to remain professional while being compassionate.

Doctoring issues:
The "doctor's dilemma" of what to tell a patient about the patient's recovery prospects.

Allowing the patient to be a partner in the healing process.

Patient issues:
The "patient's dilemma" of whether to try for the next level of recovery or remain at the existing level.

What is a "good" patient according to nurses and the patient himself?

On becoming psychologically institutionalized.

Life inside a totally paralyzed body while on a ventilator.

The importance of family, friends, and other visitors.

Illusions can be useful for mental well-being.

A look at the irrational behavior that we all have at times.

Determining the correct amount of physical therapy.

Psychological issues:
Psycho-babble vs a common sense, pragmatic method of counseling.

The harmful psychiatric method of too much, too soon.

Understanding the "demons" inside one's head and what they really are.

What it's like to die, and the "dying experience" explained medically.

Philosophical issues:
The meaning of "handicapped" and what a patient must accept.

Does altruism really exist?

Examining the "real self" and why we try to hide it.

This story is not always uplifting. It is impossible to fight for survival and mental well-being for almost three years in a hospital without experiencing tremendous highs and lows and I share them with you.

Come along and experience with me, the fears, frustrations and triumphs that unfold along the way.

Chapter 1

A Dark Omen

"Beware the Ides of March."
Julius Caesar, William Shakespeare

The paralysis began on Monday morning....
The alarm clock jolted me awake. "Damn," I muttered back at the noise. It seemed as though I had just fallen asleep after tossing and turning all night. I reached over, fumbled for the alarm button and turned it off.

Still tired, I lay back to give my body a few more minutes of rest. I wished I hadn't completely exhausted myself yesterday planting trees. I had pushed myself way too hard.

When I finally swung my legs out of bed, I noticed my toes felt numb as they touched the carpet. "Feet are still asleep," I thought without concern and turned my thoughts toward getting ready for work. After a restless night, I was groggy as I slowly walked into the bathroom, turned on the faucet, and splashed some cold water on my face.

I snapped fully awake! My fingertips were numb too. My tiredness disappeared immediately as I focused my full attention on the numbness in my fingers and toes. I wiggled my fingers. Then I wiggled my toes. Only the tips had no feeling. Everything else seemed all right so my anxiety settled down and I breathed a small sigh of relief.

"Whew, it's okay, just take a few minutes to get the feeling back," I tried to reassure myself—though I felt a strange, deep-down uneasiness that something might be terribly wrong.

I forced my thoughts back to my usual morning routine, preferring not to think about the possible cause of the numbness.

"No problem. I'm in great shape," I said aloud and smiled a half-hearted smile at myself in the mirror as I began shaving.

At age forty-six, I felt in the best physical condition of my life. I had kept myself physically fit since I was a teenager with good eating habits and disciplined exercise, mainly weight lifting. Recently, I had complimented myself for losing a couple of extra pounds around my waist. My muscles were toned and my clothes felt good against them as I dressed.

I tied a Windsor knot in my tie, slipped on my sportcoat, and patted cologne on my cheeks. I took a lot of pride in dressing well. As a final touch, I carefully brushed my hair to cover the areas where it was thinning. I was self-conscious about that.

"What a beautiful day," I thought as I shut the front door behind me and took a deep breath of fresh ocean air. Though it was March, the weather in southern California was warm and clear.

I slid behind the wheel of my Cadillac, backed out of the driveway, and headed for work. I was living the good life and I knew it. I had excellent health, a nice home near the beach, and a prosperous engineering career. Everything in my life was going well and I was certain the annoying numbness would disappear later in the day.

It was the start of a new week and I needed a cup of strong coffee to get myself going. On the way to work, I always stopped for coffee at a little outdoor hamburger stand near the beach. I pulled over to the curb in front of the Beach Burger. The food service area was just large enough for Lois to cook and serve the beach crowd. A small canopy sheltered customers while they stood around eating or sat at the lone picnic table.

"Morning John," Lois greeted me with a smile. She always looked nice, her hair neatly pulled back. She automatically poured my coffee into a foam cup to go.

"Boy, I wish I was heading for the beach myself," I said to the bronzed teenager in trunks standing next to me.

"Yeah, the swells are really full," he surfer-talked.

Lois handed me my coffee and I handed her a couple of bucks.

"See ya," I said to Lois and the surfer as I left. Back in my car, I gently placed the coffee in the holder and turned the key in the ignition. The big engine roared to life. In minutes, I was driving along the Pacific shore, breathing the fresh sea air.

Young children were walking to school with their backpacks filled with books and lunches. Older boys were out surfing, their black wetsuits glistening in the morning sun. I

6

wondered why they weren't on their way to school too.

Cruising along the ocean drive, I sipped my coffee and turned some soothing music on the radio. A slight adjustment reclined my seat into a comfortable position.

"This is going to be a good day." I cheerfully said to myself. "That numbness should be gone once I get busy."

I casually drove the few miles through Redondo, Hermosa and Manhattan Beaches. It was a clear morning. The curving, creamy shoreline of the whole bay was visible and I could see the white buildings of Santa Monica far off in the distance ahead.

Out to sea, the shape of Catalina Island loomed on the horizon like some huge, gray ship. Dozens of white sailboats were leisurely cutting through the water just beyond the surf.

When I reached Grand Avenue, I turned inland, pointing my Cad's hoodwreath toward the city of El Segundo. A couple of miles ahead was Western Industries where I was on contract as a manufacturing engineer. I contracted with various aerospace companies in the Los Angeles area, but I liked this assignment best because it was near the ocean and out of the smoggy downtown area. I had worked there for over two years.

I turned into the parking lot, found my space, and switched off the engine. I walked into the engineering department's side entrance and greeted the six other engineers as I settled down at my desk. After unpacking my attaché case, I got right to work. There was a lot to do.

It was a typical Monday morning, filled with all those work problems that seemed important at the time. My mind was busily occupied and I shut out thinking about the numbness.

At noon, I grabbed a sandwich and coffee off the lunch truck and took a short break. After eating, I walked down the hall to the office of a good friend. Hugh Whelpton was a bright guy and I thought I'd get his opinion on the lack of sensation in my fingers and toes.

I tried to sound casual as I explained my condition. Hugh listened intently without interrupting. After I finished, he smiled, shrugged his shoulders, and said the feeling would probably return soon. We both laughed it off as nothing serious—but neither of us was sure of that.

Another good friend advised me to take the day off and get some rest. It was good advice, but I foolishly ignored it and stayed at work.

The rest of the day went by without event. At five o'clock, I packed my attaché case and left. Just as I had predicted, it turned out to be a very nice day even though the numbness hadn't changed.

I knew I should go straight home and get some rest, but I was trying to keep my mind occupied to avoid thinking about the numbness. I decided to shop for a pair of shoes for my teenage son, Chris, who lived nearby with my ex-wife. I spent an hour in the shopping mall till I found the right ones. Afterward, I drove to the supermarket and did my weekly grocery shopping.

It had been a very full day. I was extremely tired and knew I shouldn't have pushed myself so hard. The numbness in my fingers and toes probably wasn't helped by draining away my energy. It was dark by the time I pulled into my driveway. I could hear my dog's welcoming bark telling me he was glad I was home.

Spunky was tied up all day so I always set him free when I got home. He whined softly, licked my hand and squirmed with anticipation, making it difficult for me to unhook his leash—especially with my numb fingers. Once free, he took off in a wild dash around the yard. I chased him for a few minutes, playing the game we played every night. After circling the backyard a few times, he let me catch him. I rolled him over and roughed him up while he pretended to bite me.

That little playtime sapped my last bit of energy. I was breathing hard. I checked my hands and feet. Nothing had changed. No more, no less. I was disappointed the feeling hadn't returned after a whole day.

I told myself, "Oh well, I'll get a good night's sleep and tomorrow I'll be back to normal"—but serious doubts remained in the back of my mind....

Chapter 2

Decision Time

"Delay always breeds danger."
Don Quixote, Miguel de Cervantes Saavedra

The alarm rang. Tuesday morning. I awoke instantly and immediately checked my hands and feet. They were still numb...

"Damn! What's going on?"

I walked into the bathroom to begin my morning routine. While brushing my teeth, I noticed I couldn't get a good grip on the toothbrush. My hands were clumsy and I couldn't control them. The numbness had spread to my hands! Now there was no use fooling myself by pretending the problem would go away. Even in this early stage of paralysis, I knew that numbness in the extremities could be a symptom of a serious problem. Somehow I managed to fumble through showering and shaving, but I knew that the concerns I had yesterday were real.

However, I've always had grace under pressure, so I didn't panic. Instead, I focused on getting ready for work and followed my normal routine. After fumbling with my clumsy hands, I managed to put on my clothes, tie my tie, and slip on my suitcoat.

As I closed the front door behind me, I could see the morning sky was clear and blue with cottony clouds. Spunky was barking goodbye as I backed out of the driveway. I pointed the Cad's hood-wreath toward the Beach Burger for my morning coffee.

The March air was fresh and crisp coming through the open car window. I tried to take a deep breath—but I couldn't. I tried again but my chest muscles would only expand enough to allow me a shallow breath. I kept trying but I couldn't get a full breath no matter how hard I tried.

I knew what was happening. My chest muscles were partially paralyzed too. This was serious. The numbness in my fingers and toes was alarming, but not being able to breathe was life threatening!

At this point in time I didn't doubt the seriousness of my condition, but I wasn't quite ready to accept the worst. Illness was a stranger to me; I had been extremely healthy my whole life. I had always been a positive thinker and believed I could fight off any problem with the right attitude.

I drove straight to work, not stopping for coffee. I didn't remember the drive to work at all. No ocean, no surfers, no sailboats. Only one thing was on my mind—the creeping numbness. My mind was trying desperately to figure out what was slowly taking control of my body.

Before I knew it, I was at Western Industries, walking with effort across the parking lot. My once strong legs felt weak and rubbery. I knew this was more than mere numbness, it was a form of paralysis that was moving fast. No doubts remained in my mind. I was in deep trouble!

"Good morning Pete. Morning Bill," I forced a smile as I unpacked my briefcase. I didn't say anything further. I was glad everyone was too busy to start a conversation because I wasn't in the mood for smalltalk.

During the morning hours I sat quietly at my desk, conserving my energy, not wanting anyone to know of my deteriorating condition.

I finished typing a report on the computer, but typing was slow and difficult. I was barely able to finish a single page before my hands and arms became limp from exhaustion.

I had to talk to someone. Bill was sitting at his desk a few feet away.

"Hi Bill." He stopped what he was doing and gave me his attention.

"You know, I've got a little problem," I smiled and tried to sound casual. "I handled some chemicals last Sunday and now my hands and feet are a little numb. I think the stuff that caused it was insecticide."

Bill joked back, "Sure, That's what insecticide does to bugs too. It numbs 'em till they're dead." Of course, he didn't realize the seriousness of what he had said.

Once I began talking, the words began to cascade out of me like a fountain.

"Bill, two days ago, on Sunday, I felt really great. First thing in the morning I worked out with my weights, had a nice breakfast, and decided to plant a few trees that I had bought at the nursery the day before."

Bill seemed interested so I kept talking.

"I've been landscaping the front of my house for the past few weeks. I had this huge, old pine tree out front and its trunk was slowly splitting down the middle from the weight of its heavy branches. As much as I hated to have that wonderful old tree cut down, I had no choice. It was splitting all apart and couldn't be saved, so I had it removed."

Bill didn't interrupt. He let me ramble on without making any comments.

"In order to plant my new trees, Bill, I had to dig out the hundreds of roots from the old pine tree that spread like tentacles under my whole front lawn. It was tough work. Using a shovel, a hatchet, and a long crowbar, I dug, chopped, and pried out most of the roots one by one."

Bill seemed absorbed by my story.

"After a few hours of this hard work, I put down my tools to take a short rest. My energy was draining but I wanted to clear out enough roots so I could plant the trees before dark.

"I needed a smaller shovel that was in the trunk of my car. After opening the trunk lid, I saw the carpeting was soaked with water. It had rained the night before and the rain must have leaked through the trunklid seal. I removed the spare tire, tools, and other stuff so I could pull out the carpeting.

"I twisted the small carpet to wring out the rainwater and immediately felt a strange sensation in my hands. It was the same feeling you get when you handle a volatile liquid like gasoline and the rapid evaporation causes a cool, tingling feeling. At the same time that I felt the tingling sensation in my hands, I tasted a strong acid taste in my mouth that was hot and bitter.

"I dropped the carpet in surprise. I figured the rainwater must have mixed with some chemicals that had spilled in the trunk. Whatever this mixture was, it had been absorbed instantly through the pores of my hands and went throughout my body immediately.

"At the time Bill, I wasn't especially alarmed. I merely wondered what was in the carpet. In the past week, I had been doing different projects around the house and had hauled a variety of things in the trunk. It could have been insecticide, fertilizer, paint thinner, auto fluids, or any combination of them. There was just no way to pinpoint the exact chemicals that were racing through my body.

"I shrugged it off and picked up the carpet again to finish wringing it out. I got the same sensation, but I ignored it. Then I went back to digging and chopping. However, I noticed that whenever I stopped working to get a drink of water or a soda, my mouth tasted a hot, strong chemical taste. Everything tasted metallic and hot. My body wasn't neutralizing the toxic stuff in my bloodstream. Still, I wasn't alarmed.

"It was sundown when I finished digging and planting the cypress trees in the front lawn and along the driveway. Boy, was I tired. My body had told me to stop working hours ago, but I wanted to finish so I pushed myself to the point of exhaustion. I can't remember ever being that tired before. I wanted to sweep the debris off the driveway and put away the tools, but I didn't have the energy. I went straight to bed.

"Bill, have you ever been so tired that you couldn't sleep?"

He nodded he had.

I continued, "That night I tossed and turned without ever really falling asleep. It was a miserable night and I cursed myself for pushing myself so hard—especially with the unknown chemicals in my system.

"Yesterday I only had numbness in my fingers and toes, but today my legs and breathing are affected. I hope it's nothing serious, but you never know."

Bill answered sincerely, "I hope it isn't either John."

I told him, "Don't mention this to anyone. It may turn out to be nothing and I'd feel foolish."

He promised not to say anything.

Later that morning I was passing Hugh's office and decided to let him know what my condition was today. He was a positive thinker and just might give me the helpful reassurance that I needed. At a time like this, I needed someone to come up with a magical solution.

"Hi Hugh," I greeted half-heartedly.

"Remember yesterday when I mentioned I had some numbness in my fingers and toes? Today it's worse. I think I'm in a bit of trouble."

It was time to admit I had a serious problem. I sat down and proceeded to repeat the whole story to Hugh. He listened attentively, not saying a word. When I finished, there was a long, awkward silence. He had no magical solution. No words of wisdom. What could he say? He and I both knew my situation couldn't be talked away with light conversation. I smiled a mirthless smile as I left his office.

It was lunchtime. I needed something to lift my spirits so I drove to the nearby beach. I stopped in a coffee shop in Manhattan Beach where the food was good and the young waitresses all wore shorts and tanktops.

The roastbeef sandwich was tasty, but swallowing was difficult. My throat muscles couldn't push the food down very well and the sandwich seemed to stick in my throat, dry and heavy. I could get only half of it down before I gave up trying.

I knew the time had come to do something; I couldn't ignore the problem anymore. I drove back to Western Industries and went straight to the project engineer's office. He and I were scheduled to visit a vendor to discuss some production problems.

"Pete, I'll have to pass on our trip," I said with a smile, trying to cover my true feelings. "I'm not feeling well and I'm going home to rest. Sorry."

"I understand." he answered. "We'll do it tomorrow. Take care."

When I started my car's engine, I debated whether to go home and rest or go to the hospital and get a doctor's opinion of what was happening to me. I found myself driving toward home. I was in a state of denial, still not quite wanting to admit the severity of the problem?

As I drove along the ocean, I tried to reason it out. "Look, John. Why not go to the hospital? If it's nothing, fine. If it *is* something, it's better to know."

I had never before avoided facing my problems and I didn't intend to start now. The Cad seemed to make a U-turn without my conscious effort, heading for the Veterans Hospital. After driving a few miles, I was on the freeway. Twenty miles later, I arrived at the VA hospital's parking lot.

I was feeling weaker, but I knew I should take the trunk carpet with me in case the doctor wanted to examine it for toxicity. It was a struggle to push the spare tire and tools aside in order to slide out the carpet, but somehow I managed. I put the carpet in a plastic trash bag because I didn't dare handle it anymore. The short walk to the emergency admissions desk felt like a mile.

As I spoke to the admissions nurse, my speech was now thick and slurred. I apologized for my speech, explaining it was part of the problem that I wanted to see a doctor about. I filled out the forms, writing in great detail about the carpet and the chemicals in it that might be causing my problem.

When I finished filling out the forms, the admissions nurse directed me to the waiting room.

While I sat quietly in the waiting room, my mind was spinning and tumbling like a drunken acrobat. What was causing the paralysis? Would the doctor be able to stop its advance? Was I dying?

My churning thoughts were interrupted by a nurse calling my name and my attention immediately shifted back to the present.

I went into the examining room. The young doctor must have been a third-year medical student because he was superficial in his examination. He completely dismissed my story about handling the toxic carpet and didn't even want to see it. A brief tap on my knees with a rubber mallet for reflex action seemed to satisfy him that I didn't have a medical problem.

He said with indifference, "You've worked too hard today and you're just tired. Go home and get some rest. If the weakness continues, come back in a couple of days."

I was tempted to say, "Let me see a neurologist." However, I felt so relieved that a doctor had told me I was all right, I thankfully left for home. I still wanted to believe my condition wasn't critical and might somehow go away.

I pulled into my driveway around five o'clock. Spunky was barking, wanting me to untie him and chase him around the backyard. I didn't. I was too weak to play our usual game of tag. Instead, I went inside the house and lay down on the sofa.

I could feel my body slowly becoming weaker and weaker as the strength oozed out of me. I didn't know whether to call someone for help or wait and see what happened next? I knew if I waited too long that I might not have the strength to use the phone.

At around six o'clock, I decided to call for help. It was time to either make a call or risk dying all alone while lying on the sofa. Time was not on my side. I managed to pick up the phone, and with almost useless fingers, tapped in my ex-wife's number. I heard the phone ring. Charlene was usually not home at this time. It rang a second and third time.

"Hello," I heard her soft voice say. (This was the first in a series of lucky breaks).

"Hi Charlene, this is John." I tried to keep my voice cheerful. "I've got a problem. I don't know why, but my body is slowly going numb. I can barely move my arms and legs, and I'm having trouble breathing. I'd appreciate it if you and Chris would come over and help me get to Fullster Hospital."

Fullster was the closest hospital and I didn't want to drive to the VA hospital again unless I needed to be hospitalized. I thought it was too soon for that.

She didn't ask any questions. "We'll be right over."

Charlene and Chris arrived in ten minutes and we immediately left for the hospital. My son was only fifteen years old, but he was strong and able to support me well enough to get into Charlene's little VW.

Not one word was spoken on the way to the nearby hospital. Chris helped me into the admissions office where the desk clerk handed me the forms to fill out. A male nurse then sat me in a wheelchair and wheeled me into an examining room. He had to help me unzip my pants so I could give a urine sample. My hands were barely able to complete the task.

A doctor soon came in. Through rubbery lips, I fully explained my problem. He took a blood sample and left the room with both samples. I sat alone waiting anxiously for the results of the analyses, hoping they would show the toxicity and I'd be given an antidote.

The doctor returned in about twenty minutes with the computer printout.

"John, I'm happy to say the tests were all negative." However, he didn't tell me what he had tested for.

He handed me the business card of a staff neurologist and told me to call him in the morning if my condition didn't improve. Neither of us realized that I was dying by inches and could not last till morning. This was the second misdiagnosis of the day.

As we drove home, I had mixed emotions. Once again, I felt relieved that a doctor had examined me and told me I was okay, but I still had no answers for my deteriorating condition. At this point, I still wasn't ready to panic because the inner strength and positive attitude I had developed during my lifetime were keeping my spirits up.

I planned my next step. Since my paralysis was not considered critical, I decided to get some rest before I saw the neurologist in the morning. However, I wanted to be near help if I needed it, so I asked Charlene if I could sleep on her sofa-bed till morning. She agreed.

We drove to her house and Chris helped me walk in. As she prepared the sofa-bed for me, I kept thinking, "This is not really happening."

Everything seemed surreal, as if it was all happening to someone else and I was merely watching the drama unfold. It was my mind's way of shutting out the terrible reality so I could mentally adjust to the problem in digestible bits, one small piece at a time.

I kept my clothes on and lay on top of the covers. Charlene turned off the lights.

I hadn't taken a deep breath since yesterday. For many minutes, I debated with myself, "Should I fall asleep? What if I never wake up?" My mind was spinning. With my thoughts rambling, I drifted off into a half-sleep.

I suddenly jerked awake. At that moment, I made a critical decision. I decided not to wait until morning to go to the hospital. The paralysis was happening too rapidly.

Charlene was asleep in the next room and Chris was in another bedroom.

I called out in the dark, "Charlene." My voice was so weak it surprised me.

"Charlene!" I forced myself to yell as loudly as possible, but it was still barely audible.

The thought crossed my mind, "What if she's in a deep sleep and doesn't even hear me? I can't get up by myself and I'll die right here when my breathing fails."

"Charlene!" I tried once more and waited.

She came into the room. She said she hadn't been sleeping and heard my first call for help but had to dress. (This was my second critical piece of luck. If she had not heard me, I was too weak to call out louder).

I asked her in a telling way, "Should we wait until morning or go to the VA hospital now?"

She said what I wanted to hear, "Let's go now."

Charlene went to get Chris and they came into the room a few minutes later, ready to go. I was much weaker now and wasn't sure whether my son would be able to support me to walk.

"I can't help you much, son," I apologized with slurred speech. I half walked and Chris half carried me to Charlene's car and helped me into the passenger's seat.

Charlene's VW had been having starting problems and sometimes the key would not turn in the ignition. If it happened now, I could be in trouble because I didn't know how long I could breathe while waiting for a road-service truck—or an ambulance.

She inserted the key, turned it, and the little engine came alive. (My third piece of luck).

Charlene didn't turn on the radio and we sat quietly as she drove through the deserted, late-night streets leading to the freeway. We were all in a tense mood, not sure what lay ahead.

The freeway was also clear of traffic at this late hour. Charlene drove at the maximum speed limit so I knew it would take almost a half-hour to get to the hospital. I sat near the window, watching neon signs of stores pass by. My breathing was difficult but not too uncomfortable so I leaned back and tried to relax. The rhythm of the engine and freeway lights methodically passing by lulled me into a dreamy state of semiconsciousness. My mind drifted....

Soon the large, white VA Hospital building appeared and brought me back to reality. I directed Charlene to turn off the freeway and follow the road leading to the emergency entrance. We stopped by the curb. Charlene got out and opened my car door. I tried to swing my legs out but couldn't move them, so I told Chris to fetch a wheelchair from inside. He came back with one immediately and he and Charlene helped ease me from the front seat onto the wheelchair. I was in bad shape. My arms and legs flopped uselessly. My breathing was now dangerously shallow.

The nurse at the admissions desk saw my condition and directed us straight to the emergency room. Two young student-doctors who looked like they hadn't slept in days, sprang into action. With Chris' help, they lifted me onto the examining gurney. As I tried to tell them my problem through numb lips, they were stripping off my clothes and slipping a hospital gown on me. One doctor shined an ophthalmoscope in my eyes while the other was pumping up a blood pressure cuff on my arm.

Things were happening fast now. I could barely breathe.

I gasped, "I can't breathe! I can't breathe!" I was in mortal danger.

One doctor hurried to the phone, calling the intensive care unit to prepare for me.

"I need air!" I gasped, "Air!"

They quickly wheeled me out of the emergency room and down the hall. Lying on my back, I watched the fluorescent lights pass overhead. We stopped at an elevator. Waited. Doors opened. Up. Stop. Off. Down two hallways. Through swinging doors. Past beds with patients and into a small, one-bed cubicle. I was in an isolation booth in the Intensive Care Unit.

Two doctors and four nurses surrounded my gurney. Many hands lifted me up and onto the bed.

"I can't breathe!," I wheezed again and again.

Neither paralysis nor pain mattered now. All I wanted was air. Precious air. I needed air!

A doctor attempted to insert a naso-endotracheal tube. I automatically fought it with all the strength I had left. I needed the breathing tube, but jamming a foreign object in my nose caused me to gag and instinctively resist. My body was just strong enough to interfere with his efforts.

"We'd better give him five milligrams of valium," I heard someone say. They knew they had to calm me down in order to thread the air tube into my trachea.

The level of action around me was intense. Nurses and doctors were all moving at top speed to keep me alive. Two held me down, another gave me a shot, and one doctor was shoving a laryngoscope into my mouth to hold down my tongue while the other doctor was trying to snake the endotracheal tube past my tongue. Everyone was talking at once.

I couldn't swallow to help them, but somehow they threaded the tube into my trachea and immediately connected it to a ventilator.

I was now intubated and had made it to this life-saving ventilator with no time to spare! (This was my final piece of luck for the evening).

Heart monitoring wires were taped to my chest for signs of tachycardia and my heart rate was displayed on a digital readout unit on a shelf above my head. A blood gas sample was drawn to set the ventilator's oxygen output. Suspecting my trauma was due to Guillain Barré Syndrome, I was given 100 units of ACTH.

That was all the staff could do at the moment. I was stabilized. Everyone left the isolation booth.

I was alone, completely alone. Now the struggle for life would begin. It would be a long battle, filled with trauma, pain, misery.

Chapter 3

One Is A Lonely Number

"Alone, alone,—all, all alone."
The Ancient Mariner,
Samuel Taylor Coleridge

The small isolation booth was just large enough for my bed and medical equipment. I was being isolated until they knew whether or not I had a contagious disease. The door was kept closed. I felt abandoned. I was totally helpless in this unfamiliar place with an unknown force taking total control of my body. This strange, frightening place was ominously silent except for the gentle swooshing sound of the ventilator bellows as it rose and fell. Swoosh, pause, swoosh, pause, swoosh... The machine was rhythmically pumping 700 milliliters of 30% oxygenated air, 13 times a minute, into my nearly lifeless lungs which could barely assist the ventilator.

My enclosed booth was in the corner of the room. There were windows to the outside on my left and behind my bed, but they were too high for me to see out. The interior window on the right side of my booth faced the ward and I could see the activity on the ward when lying on my right side. There were five beds outside my booth, side by side, with the nurses sitting at their open station midway down.

I was alert, aware of every inch of my body. I could feel my muscles becoming more and more useless. The ventilator was not the wonderful provider of air that I expected. Instead of large puffs of refreshing oxygen, the ventilator was set at the minimal level to keep me alive. I barely felt the oxygen going into me and I worried I would suffocate at any minute. I had to fight off panicking because I knew my mind could play tricks on me and make me feel short of air even if I wasn't.

A lot of things were happening inside my body. Since my lungs were only being partially inflated, the lower sacs were beginning to fill with fluids. My inability to move and to swallow left my body incapable of dealing with all the internal secretions. Saliva was flowing out of my mouth and pooling on the pillow.

Meanwhile, the toxicity in my blood had reached my internal organs and the battle between the toxins and my immune system was raging. My whole body was weak and feverish.

This was my world now. Alone in a small isolation booth, feverish, feeling suffocated from lack of oxygen, and choking on my own fluids. The paralysis continued to spread and I was now almost totally paralyzed. Though my motor nerves were useless, my sensory nerves were functioning perfectly. I could feel everything even though I couldn't move. My mind was alert and aware of everything that was happening, but I was a prisoner inside my lifeless body.

I felt near death. Was this really happening to me? Why were the nurses leaving me all alone in this closed room? Couldn't they see I was choking? I desperately needed someone near me to give me a feeling of security, to know I wasn't abandoned and left to die alone.

A long, slow hour passed. Finally, a nurse came into my booth to check my vital signs. After she checked my blood pressure, pulse, and temperature, she left and closed the door behind her. The doctors still didn't know what was causing my paralysis, so I would be monitored every two hours.

It was the middle of the night. The lights had been dimmed and everything was quiet except for the whooshing sound of the ventilator bellows.

A large, ominous looking woman in a white coat entered my room. She didn't say a word as she began her work. In my helpless state, she was extremely intimidating because I had no idea what she was going to do. When I saw her check out the ventilator, I recognized she must be a respiratory therapist.

She disconnected the ventilator hose from my endo-tracheal tube. I was without air and started to panic! The RT stuck a respirometer between my lips and told me, "Press your lips together and hold this." I tried to grip the mouthpiece with my lips but I had no lip strength at all. She quickly connected the gauge to the endotracheal tube and said, "Inhale as much as you can and slowly blow it all out." She waited a few seconds, and muttered, "Nothing." The needle on the dial to

21

measure my exhaled air for vital capacity hadn't moved.

I was still disconnected from the ventilator and my anxiety was building. Next, she connected a pressure gauge to my endotracheal tube and told me, "Exhale, then inhale as much as you can." The gauge's needle to measure my negative inspiration pressure also didn't move. She tried again with the same results. My paralyzed muscles couldn't expand my chest enough to register a reading. I could feel my temperature rising from the lack of oxygen.

She finally gave up and reconnected my endotracheal tube to the ventilator. During this procedure, I had been without oxygen for only a minute, but it seemed much longer. Nothing had ever struck more fear into me than not being able to breathe. At that point, I realized just how vulnerable I was. Anyone could enter my room and do whatever they wanted to do to me. I could not speak to complain or move my arms to resist. My life was at the mercy of others.

The hours of that first night passed slowly. I was awake every second. I felt that I was slowly dying and didn't know why. What did I have? I didn't know if the paralysis was due to the toxic chemicals I had handled, or some other disease that I didn't even know about. I kept trying to understand what was going on inside my deteriorating body.

Finally, the morning sun came shining through the two outside windows and my room began to lighten. Morning brought a flurry of activity on the ward. I could see all the action through the window of my booth. The dayshift doctors came on duty and made their rounds. The dayshift nurses began giving medications to wakened patients. Kitchen helpers brought breakfast trays for patients who were able to eat and nurses helped those who couldn't feed themselves. Respiratory therapists came to service the ventilators. X-ray technicians wheeled in a portable machine to take photos. Physical therapists arrived to give range of motion. People seemed to be moving in all directions.

No one was allowed in my isolation booth unless they had a required duty to perform. My diagnosis was still undetermined so they weren't taking any chances of exposing anyone to a possibly contagious disease. After an hour, one of the six nurses on duty in the unit came to check my vital signs. She didn't say a word to me throughout the check.

Soon after, a staff doctor and an entourage of third-year medical students came on grand rounds. The older, balding doctor picked up my chart as he introduced himself.

"Good morning, Mr. Sueta. My name is Dr. Hanson. I'm chief of neurology."

The young doctors-in-training said nothing as they listened attentively to their mentor.

"John, try moving your fingers."

I tried but couldn't.

"That's okay John. Try moving your toes."

I couldn't.

Putting down my chart, Dr. Hanson took a small needle out of his pocket.

"I know you can't answer, so blink your eyes if you feel anything."

He pricked up and down my arms. I blinked with each stick. He continued sticking my legs, the soles of my feet, my chest, and my face. I blinked every time he touched me. My sensory nerves were all working fine.

At that point, Dr. Hanson spoke to his young students and discussed my case with them as if I wasn't even in the room.

"Mr. Sueta's sensory nerves are obviously intact, but his motor nerves have been affected. Until we get the results of his blood test and do a lumbar puncture, we won't know if his symptoms point to postdiphtheritic neuritis, multiple sclerosis, porphyria, mycoplasma, acute demylenating polyneuropathy, botulism, chronic or acute idiopathology."

It sounded like a verbal autopsy. I never could understand why doctors talked so openly about a patient's condition while in the patient's presence. But, at the same time, I was glad to know what the possibilities were. I wanted to know as much as I could about the disease that was invading my body. Though I didn't understand everything he listed as possible causes, I did recognize a few. None of them sounded good.

Before leaving, Dr. Hanson smiled and said in a loud, positive voice, "John, you'll be walking out of the hospital within thirty days."

(This was the third misdiagnosis in the past twenty-four hours).

23

Wow! I was ecstatic. I couldn't yell or even smile, but I had a great feeling of relief and joy. The paralysis had come on suddenly and would go away just as quickly. Dr. Hanson's analysis indicated my recovery would turn a sharp corner soon and I'd be on my feet again, feeling like my old self.

My exhilaration ended when the nurse came in with a cart full of bottles, syringes, and tubes. She explained that she was going to put an intravenous tube in my arm. The stick was fairly painless and she attached an IV bag. All went well.

Charlene and Chris came into the room. They had stayed all night in the visitors' waiting room and they looked exhausted. They were as troubled as I was, not knowing what my condition was.

My appearance didn't help. I looked a mess but I was happy to see friendly faces in this sea of strangers. I had the IV in my arm, heart-monitoring electrodes taped to my chest, and the ventilator tube stuck in my nose, Fluids were coming out of my mouth and nose, gagging me. I wanted to ask them to wipe it away, but how could I?

Chris seemed to understand. He picked up the suctioning catheter, figured out how to turn on the vacuum, and suctioned the fluids around my nose and mouth that were gagging my minimal breathing. It helped.

Charlene and Chris were tired and uncomfortable. They didn't know what to say and I could only lie there in silence. Except for limited eye expressions, I had no way to communicate. After a few minutes, Charlene said she had to leave for work, but they would be back to see me as soon as possible.

When they left, I felt alone and helpless again. My life was back in the hands of strangers with no one to speak for me. Because of my vulnerability, the hospital seemed a hostile place.

Meanwhile, the paralysis continued to attack my body, inch by inch. It reached its worst point that day when I could only blink my eyes, move my lower jaw, and somewhat control my bladder and bowels. That was the only motor control I had left. All other movement was gone. Internally, my liver was inflamed and I was running a high fever. My body was a lifeless, uncontrollable mass of limp flesh. The fact my mind was fully alert and I had total sensory feeling made my plight even worse because I was aware of everything and felt every pain.

Blood pressure, pulse rate, breathing, and temperature checks were taken every two hours. The worst check was the arterial blood gas drawing. The ABG had to be monitored often to check the amount of oxygen and electrolytes in my blood. The samples were sent to the laboratory for computer analysis to determine the ventilator settings. Since my muscles were becoming more and more flaccid, it was becoming progressively more difficult to find my arteries for blood drawing as they slowly sank deeper into my soft flesh. I couldn't make a fist to help expose them, so each blood drawing took a lot of probing and many painful needle sticks.

In the afternoon, a young doctor came into the booth and introduced himself. He was probably an intern.

"Good afternoon John. I'm Dr. Singer and I'll be your doctor. I don't have much to tell you yet. We won't be sure what your problem is until all our tests are completed. As soon I get the results, I'll let you know. Until then, just hang in there.

"I realize that tube in your nose is uncomfortable so we're thinking of scheduling you for a tracheotomy. It's an operation where we put a breathing tube directly into your throat and get rid of that tube in your nose. Once you have the tracheostomy tube, you'll be more comfortable and be able to breathe better. Would you like that? Blink your eyes once for `yes' or twice for `no.' "

The thought of breathing easier gave me a spark of hope. As it was now, I felt critically short of oxygen and worried I'd either suffocate or suffer brain damage from lack of oxygen. Why wasn't the ventilator pumping big blasts of air into my hungry lungs instead of sending small wisps of air that were barely enough to keep me alive?

Dr. Singer called a nurse to witness my eye-blink approval and said, "I'll schedule the operation for next Monday." He made a note of it and left.

Today was only Wednesday. Could I live in this condition for five days? I wasn't sure. The fluids were filling my nose, mouth, and lungs almost as soon as they were suctioned.

25

The nurse assigned to me that day came into the booth and stood by my bed, staring down at me. I pleaded as best I could with my eyes for suctioning—or anything. I just needed someone near me. I didn't want to be left all alone in this isolated room with no one to help me if I stopped breathing or had cardiac arrest. I needed the reassurance of human contact. She left.

The late afternoon passed slowly and turned into night. At ten o'clock, the lights on the ward were dimmed, TVs turned off, and it was time for patients to sleep. My small cubicle was deathly quiet except for the sound of the ventilator bellows hissing open and closed. I lay there, watching the bellows incessantly expand and contract, expand and contract....

The day's struggles had exhausted me, but the gagging and fear of suffocating wouldn't let me fall asleep. I was sure that if I fell asleep, I'd choke to death. I forced my mind to stay awake and remain alert.

I was lying on my left side facing the ventilator with pillows supporting my head, back, and between my legs. Fluids flowed out of my mouth and onto the pillow, pooling around my nose and mouth. The very small amount of air I could inhale by myself was blocked by the pooled fluid and made me gag. Each breath became more and more difficult. I was certain the ventilator was set too low. My senses were telling me that I was starving for oxygen. I fought against panicking. I knew I had to stay calm and not fight against the ventilator's rhythm.

I told myself, "Relax and breathe, relax and breathe." I kept repeating those words over and over. It took tremendous concentration to stay focused and not panic. After hours of strenuous concentration, the maddening effort began to sap my emotional and physical strength.

I was frustrated by my total helplessness and angry with the nurses for leaving me alone and not giving me the reassuring attention I needed. Why weren't they doing something—anything? I desperately needed someone standing near to assure me I wouldn't die all alone in this small, isolated booth.

My situation was like nightmares I'd had in the past when I was frozen with fear and couldn't run or scream no matter how hard I tried. In the nightmares, I was jolted awake when the fear became unbearable. Now I was having the same nightmare, only I couldn't end it by waking up—I *was* awake.

After another long, tedious hour of struggling to breathe and incessantly trying to time my breathing to match the ventilator's rhythm, I was mentally and physically exhausted. It was a battle I was losing. My fatigue and the hopelessness of my situation finally made me stop caring one way or the other whether I lived or died. I just couldn't fight anymore. I had reached the limit of my endurance.

I thought, "To hell with it, I've had enough of this misery. Living isn't worth all this." All I could think of was that I was slowly and surely suffocating to death, so why fight it? I couldn't keep resisting. I mentally broke. I quit struggling to breathe and mentally let go....

Almost immediately—I didn't know why—but I felt kind of peaceful and relaxed. My mind was clear. What a great feeling! For the first time since I entered the hospital, I felt at peace. There was no struggle to breathe. No panic. No anger. Just a warm, beautiful feeling. My mind continued to feel blissfully happy. I told myself, "Just let go, John." I felt wonderful.

But, something interrupted my pleasant aura. Somewhere in a deep recess of my mind, I believed I was dying. It felt wonderful, but was that what I really wanted? My thoughts suddenly shifted to my son Chris, who had visited me that morning. My death would bring him tremendous grief and affect his whole life.

A conflict raged within my mind of whether to continue my peaceful drifting away or to stop the journey. At that exact moment, I knew I had to make a choice. Either I could let myself continue to peacefully slip away, or else I could stop the spiral.

I made the choice. My concern for Chris was stronger than my desire to continue my pleasant but dangerous journey! I forcefully willed my mind to stop its flight into the abyss.

I was back where I started, struggling for breath to stay alive.

Chapter 4

A New Way to Communicate

"The moving finger writes; and having writ, moves on."
Rubáiyát, Omar Khayyam

I was wakened from my miserable sleep by the morning nurse coming into the booth to take my vital signs.

I turned my thoughts to my surroundings. I was lying on my right side so I could see through the window overlooking the rest of the ward. Morning brought the usual flurry of activity. Doctors were making their morning rounds and nurses were preparing patients for the breakfast trays soon to arrive. I saw Dr. Singer enter the ward and head toward my booth.

"Good morning John. I hope you're feeling better. So far we haven't been able to form a diagnosis, but we're hoping a lumbar puncture will fill in the missing pieces."

He explained how he would do the spinal tap and the possible complications. I knew the law required him to make sure I fully understood the risks. Dr. Singer had a nurse witness my eyeblink approval.

He had the necessary instruments with him so he turned me on my left side. The procedure went smoothly. Before he left, Dr. Singer promised he would let me know the results as soon as possible.

I hoped the spinal fluid would reveal the source of my paralysis and show it was not irreversible. While I waited to know the results, I tried to keep my mind occupied. I was now on my left side, so I studied the ventilator. I was familiar with this ventilator because I had a friend who worked at the Bennett Company and we had discussed how they functioned. Now one of their machines was all that stood between me and death.

The ventilator was set at 700 ml of air. Any effort I made to breathe wouldn't change the preset volume. What I didn't know was that if my effort to breathe was strong enough, the machine would respond by pumping an extra breath. However, my ability to breathe was so weak I couldn't trigger any extra breaths.

The doctor in charge of my ventilator noticed I wasn't lighting up the "assist" light, so he increased the amount of oxygen. I wasn't aware of the increase because it didn't make a noticeable difference.

Every bit of air was precious, so I tried to coordinate my shallow breathing with the machine. In order to receive the maximum volume of air, I had to be inhaling as best I could, when the bellows was collapsing and exhaling when the bellows was rising. I was glad I had an older-model ventilator with the exposed bellows because it allowed me to visually time my breathing with the bellow's rise and fall.

The rhythm of the bellow's rise and fall became my mental rhythm. I counted the seconds between the puffs of air so that I knew exactly when to breathe in harmony with the machine. Though my ability to breathe was almost zero, I had to control whatever respiration I could and not fight against the timing of the ventilator.

There was only one thing I had full control over—urinating. Since this was the only thing I had control over, it was extremely important to me. I took great satisfaction in urinating into my condom catheter and turned it into a long ritual. First I carefully prepared myself to urinate, then I slowly controlled the release of the liquid, and when I was finished, I complimented myself on my accomplishment. The control I had over urinating, as seemingly unimportant as it was, was psychologically important to me.

It was critical to my mental health to have some control in my life—any control. Without that, I was completely helpless. It was maddening to lie immobile, mentally telling my body to do things and getting no response. I needed to have something that responded to my will, no matter how small.

Only a short while ago I was a healthy, strong, independent man who didn't depend on anyone for anything. I could climb stairs two at a time, run for miles, and lift a barbell with hundreds of pounds of weights on it. Now I lay helpless, unable to move a finger.

I was completely dependent on others for everything. The hospital staff did a good job of caring for me, but they were in control of my life and I was at their mercy.

Many times I wanted to yell out in frustration, but I was voiceless. The frustration was intense. I wanted to cry from bitter helplessness, but when I teared up, my nose and throat clogged up with fluids that made me gag and choke. I didn't even have the luxury of allowing my frustrations to be let out. Satan couldn't have designed a more fiendish torture.

Inside my mind was the terrible uncertainty of what was happening to me and where it would all end. Did I have toxic poisoning? Did I have some form of polio or multiple sclerosis? Had I injured my spine digging out tree roots? I didn't know, and so far neither did any of the neurological teams of doctors who had examined me.

How long could I lie totally immobile with my lungs constantly filling up with fluids before I choked to death or my heart went into cardiac arrest?

I slept in short, uncomfortable naps. During those naps, I always dreamed I was my normal self. I was never paralyzed nor bedridden. I recalled reading about Roy Campanella, a former catcher for the Brooklyn Dodgers who was permanently confined to a wheelchair after his spine was injured in a car accident. He said that in his dreams he was always the way he was before the accident, physically active and still playing baseball.

My dreams were similar. In my dreams, I was out of the hospital and walking down streets with fine houses and beautiful lawns, talking to people who couldn't tell I had a problem. My thoughts were, "Hey, I'm breathing on my own. I'm walking. Won't the nurses be surprised when they notice I'm not in my bed?"

Another recurring dream I had was the ability to move my fingers and make a fist. It felt wonderful to curl my fingers into a closed fist. In my dreams, I kept clenching and unclenching my hands, over and over.

When I awoke, I felt joyful that I could move my hands. Still half-asleep, I tried to make a fist. Nothing. I tried again and kept trying until my mind slowly transitioned from the dream state to reality. When I became fully awake, I realized I was still paralyzed.

I silently cursed, "Damn! Damn! Damn!"

My nursing care followed a strict schedule. Nurses turned me every two hours, suctioned me when necessary, drew ABG blood to monitor my oxygen and pH levels, and stuck a new IV in my arm when it infiltrated. Since I was in isolation, I only saw staff people who were absolutely necessary for my care.

The morning of Friday the 13th arrived. I had never been very superstitious, but in my situation, every negative possibility was magnified. I hoped nothing bad would happen that day. I was actually looking forward to Monday's tracheotomy. I believed that once an air tube was inserted directly into my trachea, I would be able to breath better than through the tube in my nose. I envisioned breathing normally and was willing to suffer any pain or discomfort.

I received some good news. Three nurses came into my room and told me they were moving me into the main ICU area outside the booth. My blood tests and spinal tap had shown I did not have a communicable disease and didn't have to be isolated.

They disconnected the heart monitor wires taped to my chest. When they disconnected the ventilator, they quickly attached an AMBU bag to my endotracheal tube. They rolled my bed and IV stand into the center of the ward where they switched places with the bed that was there. The equipment was reconnected and I had a new "home."

I was not alone anymore. Outside the booth, there were five beds side by side and I was in bed No. 3 with two patients to the left of me and two patients to the right of me. There was a clock and a TV set on the wall in front of me. Most importantly, the nurses' station was not enclosed and was directly across the aisle from the foot of my bed. They could closely watch me in case of an emergency.

Each day at around five o'clock in the afternoon, my face got very hot as a fever began to fight against the disease rampaging through my body. The fevers lasted for an hour, then subsided. They continued daily despite the fact I was naked with only a sheet covering me. I didn't have blankets because even that small amount of weight on my chest interfered with my efforts to breathe. I didn't wear a hospital gown because it could twist and put pressure on my chest.

ICU's business never stopped. The intensive care unit was always bustling with activity. Nurses, doctors, respiratory therapists, X-ray technicians, food servers, chaplains, and family members came in and out all day. Visitors were allowed at any time. New patients were brought in at all hours of the day and night to replace patients being moved out into less critical care wards—or the morgue. Last night, the Code Blue Team had run in to perform heroic measures and save the man in the next bed.

My assigned nurse for the day was a lovely young Puerto Rican girl named Rosa. She had long, auburn hair, beautiful white teeth, and a sweet gentleness. I immediately liked her. I guess she liked me too because when time permitted, Rosa sat by my bed and talked to me. She said she prayed for my recovery. Whenever I needed suctioning or anything else, she was there for me.

One of the other young nurses was also attentive to my situation. She wasn't assigned to me that day, but she came to my bedside to show me something. She held a piece of cardboard upon which she had printed the alphabet in bold black letters with a felt-tip pen.

"Hi John, I'm Linda. I know you've been trying to communicate with us so I made this chart. You can spell words by blinking your eyes when I point to the right letter. Would you like to try it."

I blinked once.

She began with "A", then "B", and kept pointing until she came to "H." I blinked.

She began with "A" again. I blinked when she got to "E."

She began again with "A." I blinked at "L."

Then "L" again. Then "O."

Then I blinked "L-I-N-D-A." She was pleased and gave me a wonderful smile. This fine young nurse had gone out of her way to open up a whole new way to communicate.

I felt a tremendous surge of excitement. Until now the only way I had to communicate was by using my eyes. I widened them to express my anxiety, squinted to show I didn't understand or felt pain, or softened them when I was pleased. I stared at the nasal catheter for suctioning. I looked downward if I needed the bedpan. That limited me to the very basics.

Now I'd be able to more fully express myself.

Unfortunately, many of the staff chose not to use the alphabet board. It seemed simple, but most didn't have the time it took to slowly spell words.

Some nurses couldn't get the hang of it. They would start with "A", but when I blinked for a letter, they didn't re-start with "A" again and instead continued on from that letter. That ended in failure and frustrated both of us. With them, I tried to spell out words that didn't require backing up, such as "air" or "TV" or "first." That required a great amount of planning on my part. I kept my messages brief, with as few words as possible, resulting in a form of "pidgin English."

Some nurses were foreign born and didn't speak English well. Trying to remember the letters I had spelled out and then forming them into words confused them. At first, they tried to use the alphabet board, but gave up in frustration when things didn't go well.

However, for Rosa and those who took the time to use the alphabet board, it opened up a deeper understanding between us.

When the day shift nurses went home, the level of activity on the ward slowed down. The afternoon shift was less busy and at ten o'clock, the fluorescent lights were dimmed and the TVs turned off so patients could sleep. The only sounds were patients' coughing or moaning in pain. Unless an emergency broke the stillness, all was quiet. I dozed off.

At 2 A.M., the night nurse woke me for a bedbath by turning on the bright light above my head. Its glare burned my eyes. Since the nighshift nurses were not as busy, bedbaths were done in the middle of the night for the convenience of the staff—certainly not for mine. The air-conditioning blowing on my wet body was chilling and moving me was painful. They finished quickly. I understood how strenuous it was for nurses to physically maneuver a limp patient like me and why they tried to get it over with quickly, though roughly.

It was important to me when nurses explained beforehand what they were going to do. I appreciated knowing what was about to be done so I could mentally prepare myself. The more considerate nurses explained, "John, I'm going to change your IV, it will only take a minute," or "John, I'm going to take a blood gas sample, so relax." It meant a lot to me when they prepared me.

Chapter 5

Tracheotomy Time

"What we anticipate seldom occurs;
what we least expected generally happens."
Benjamin Disraeli (1804-1881)

The weekend passed slowly with no relief in my struggle to breathe.The days were an endless series of being examined, turned, suctioned, and injected. Charlene and Chris visited me in my new location, but the sight of all the tubes and wires sticking out of me and witnessing the miserable plight of patients nearby was disturbing, so they didn't stay long nor visit often.

I was glad no one else came to visit because it would have been too embarrassing to have others see me like this. I hadn't been shaved since entering the hospital and my hair was a matted mess. Right or wrong, I still had my vanity.

However, I did receive a get-well card signed by all the people at Western Industries. Rosa showed it to me and read the encouraging messages. They also had sent a potted plant that I cherished because a healthy, living thing on my bedside table represented life itself to me and softened the cold hospital surroundings. Rosa made sure it was carefully watered.

Monday morning arrived. It was operation day! At nine o'clock the swinging doors were pushed open by three people dressed in green surgical smocks and hats. The surgical team wheeled their gurney next to my bed. The heart monitoring electrodes and the IVAC were disconnected. An AMBU bag replaced the ventilator tube attached to my endotracheal tube and one of the team began rhythmically squeezing oxygen into my lungs.

ICU nurses came to help slide me onto the gurney. We passed through the swinging doors, rolled down the hall, and rode the elevator up two floors to a brightly lit operating room. I had no anxiety whatsoever of the impending operation. I was anxious to have it done so I could breathe better.

Two young doctors awaited my arrival. The team slid me onto the operating table. One doctor placed a rolled up towel under my shoulder blades to hyperextend my neck and immediately gave me a local anesthetic. The surgeon probed my throat with his fingers to locate the right spot. He deftly cut through the skin and trachea. As soon as my trachea was cut open, I heard the rush of air from my lungs. It sounded like a balloon being deflated.

Quickly, the naso-endotracheal tube I had been using was pulled out and a short, hard plastic tube was pushed into the neck iincision with the tip sticking out. The doctor inflated the cuff-balloon now inside my trachea to make a seal that prevented air from escaping through the hole in my neck or up the trachea. When the string was tied around my neck to hold the tracheostomy in place, the operation was complete. The AMBU bag was attached to the tracheal tube and pumping resumed. The operation had gone smoothly with no problems and no pain.

I was wheeled back to ICU and transferred back into my bed. The ventilator was reconnected and I waited in anticipation of the wonderfully deep breaths I was sure would soon be pumped into my hungry lungs.

After a few anxious minutes, I knew the worst—I couldn't breathe any better than before the operation! The reason was clear: the ventilator was still set at the minimum level. My hope of breathing comfortably was shattered. Not only had the operation not helped my breathing, but now I had a piece of hard plastic stuck in my throat that was more uncomfortable than the nasal tube.

I remembered seeing patients on ventilators in television shows and I always imagined they were receiving nice big puffs of oxygen. The reality was different. Trying to breathe on the ventilator was like trying to breathe with a wet towel covering my nose and mouth. No matter how hard I tried to breathe, I could only draw in the tiny amount of air the ventilator was set to give. With every breath, I felt I wasn't getting enough oxygen to stay alive. I had to fight against panicking because I knew anxiety would make me struggle and I'd be out of sync with the ventilator. If that happened, I could be in real trouble.

The previous night, I had watched a panicked patient fight the ventilator. The alarm beeped loudly. The more he struggled to breathe, the worse the situation became. Nurses rushed to his aid and put an AMBU bag on him as they gave him a sedative. He slowly calmed down and they were able to reconnect him to the ventilator. It was a close call.

It took tremendous mental discipline to lie there and breathe in harmony with the machine when my instincts were telling me I needed more air and I should breathe faster. I had to maintain my discipline hour after hour as I constantly watched the bellows move up and down inside the glass jar only a few feet from my face.

I was nervous when anyone—no matter who—stood by the ventilator controls. I didn't want anyone to go near it. Were they going to turn down the volume, the percentage of oxygen, or the number of breaths? Did they know what they were doing? Did they realize how hard it was for me to breathe? All I knew was that I was living on a bare minimum of oxygen and I didn't want anyone tampering with the machine.

The morning RT had reduced the oxygen content to 25% and I complained by staring at the ventilator when the respiratory doctor was near. He turned it up to 30%. Except for the visible tidal volume markings on the bellows bowl, I had no knowledge of the other settings. I was only aware of changes in the oxygen level and number of breaths settings when they affected my ability to breathe, but I didn't know what the settings were.

There were many control buttons and they had to be checked often, but too much adjusting was going on. Why were different people resetting the ventilator? Were they competent? Even if they were, mistakes could happen.

I focused all my attention on the ventilator. The machine made a small, double-pump "sigh" eight times an hour. The sigh was barely noticeable, but I could tell by the sound of the machine when it happened. It gave an extra puff of air in two short bursts, one right after the other. The total was a larger volume of air than the usual 700 ml. By timing my breathing, I could catch the whole sigh and take a slightly deeper breath. It wasn't a big difference, but even that slight amount of extra air was worth all my efforts to get it.

I looked forward to that extra puff of air every 7½ minutes. I anxiously counted the number of breaths to it. If my timing was off and I missed it, I was angry with myself. When I did catch it, I felt a short-lived "aaah." Then I had to quickly get back to counting for the next one. The clock on the wall was directly in front of me and gave me a second way to know when the sigh was due.

The ventilator was the most important thing in my miserable life. It was my lifeline. It was my obsession. I could live for weeks without food, days without water, but only a few minutes without my precious air.

My fate was in the hands of dozens of strangers, some I trusted, some I didn't. I was distrustful of almost everyone who touched the ventilator controls or disconnected me to measure my breathing or change the tubes.

The ventilator tubes were changed regularly to prevent the humidified air's accumulated condensation from entering my lungs. The cup where condensed moisture collected also had to be emptied regularly.

It took skill to disconnect the old tubes and quickly reconnect new ones. The time varied from seconds to almost a minute, depending on the RT. Being without air even for that short time was frightening. One morning, a fumbling respiratory therapist had me disconnected so long, I had a bowel movement caused by either the lack of oxygen or my fear. I wasn't sure which.

Each morning, I was either relieved or uneasy, depending on which respiratory therapist came through the door to service my ventilator. There was one RT I trusted because of his obvious competence. Pete could disconnect me, change the tubes, and reconnect me so quickly I didn't miss a breath. It was becoming easier for me to recognize competent staff.

The doctor in charge of my ventilation was also someone I had faith in. Dr. Marshall was a tall, well-built man about thirty-five years old. He had an aura of competence. Some people exude it. I listened attentively to the conversations between him and the respiratory therapists to learn as much as I could about what they were doing. Most of the time they spoke too softly for me to hear because they thought I was too preoccupied with the ventilator. Of course I was preoccupied with it, it was all that stood between me and suffocating to death. When you can't breathe, nothing else matters!

In addition to the problem of too many people adjusting the ventilator settings, there was a design flaw with the ventilator's connection to my tracheostomy. When the tubes were changed, the output end of the new tube was slipped over the nipple of the device in my throat. The only thing that kept it connected was the friction of the ventilator tube slipping over the nipple. Possibly It was made without a locking mechanism so nurses could easily disconnect it for suctioning and reconnect it and not cause harm to the surrounding tissue by forcing it off and on.

Obviously, no two were exactly alike, so the connection was not always a good fit. Some fit snugly and stayed securely connected and some fit loosely and could pop off as the ventilator's air pressure built up. If that happened, I was disconnected from the ventilator and an alarm sounded after a ten second delay.

Whenever the air hose popped off, I waited anxiously, counting the ten seconds until the alarm sounded and a nurse hurried over to reconnect it. I would only miss a breath or two, but I couldn't understand why a life-support machine had a sloppy connector that could pop off at any time. Why wasn't there a locking mechanism? I believed that one day an RT would forget to reset the alarm after turning it off temporarily to change tubes or clean the glass bowl. If the tube popped off with the alarm switched off, no one would know I was suffocating. Why wasn't the alarm's on-off switch foolproof? I was sure some hospitals had a better system, but this is what I had.

Another alarm I hated to hear was my IVAC machine. The beeping signaled something was blocking the flow of fluid. It meant IV fluid was infiltrating into the nearby tissue and the location of the needle had to be changed, requiring many painful sticks until a vein was found. I learned to dread the sound of the IV beeper.

I was also stuck twice a day with injections of 5000 units of Heparin. Since I was completely immobile, the doctors wanted to prevent my blood from forming clots. The Heparin was injected into my abdominal area and the skin soon hardened, making it difficult for the nurses to find a soft area to use.

Despite receiving frequent suctioning, I had ongoing bilateral pneumonia and atelectasis. The pneumonia contributed to my daily fevers. One evening my temperature spiked to 103 degrees and the night duty doctor was summoned. He suctioned my lungs and extracted a large amount of mucus.

Overhearing the doctors discussing my pneumonia, I surmised they believed it was due to the accumulation of fluids from my shallow breathing and lying immobile. But, in my layman's mind, I thought the pneumonia might be due to fluids seeping past an under-inflated tracheal cuff. Without a gag reflex, I imagined mouth fluids entering my trachea and bypassing a leaky cuff. Another possibility I imagined was small pools of humidified air condensing in the ventilator's tubing and directly entering my trach tube—though I didn't know how it could get there. My mind conjured up different scenarios for my pneumonia, some likely and some far-fetched.

Lying immobile all day, I spent long hours studying things around me. I looked up at the heart monitor on the shelf above my head and could read the numbers. The electrodes taped to my chest to detect tachycardia and dysrhythmia were connected to it and the digital readout registered my constantly changing heart rate. Whenever my heart rate seemed too high, I tried to relax and get it below the tachycardia level of 100. As I relaxed, I watched it change to 105, 104, 103, 102, 101, 100, 99. I could break 100 for a few seconds, but the rate averaged around 110. I constantly worried my heart couldn't keep pumping at such a high rate indefinitely and would ultimately go into cardiac arrest.

Relaxing to lower my heartrate was also a good biofeedback method to help deal with my anxiety. Lowering my heartrate—even to such a minor degree—gave me something I had some control over. I needed every bit of control I could manage to counteract my feelings of utter helplessness.

On the amusing side, I was sure my heartrate increased a little whenever any of the attractive young nurses walked past in the aisle along the foot of the beds. ICU was blessed with a half dozen pretty, young nurses. Many times I noticed older men in the beds next to me who were barely alive, feebly turn their heads to stare at the young nurses. It was humorous to see how men's fantasies were still active, no matter how sick they were.

Surprisingly, I felt no embarrassment when the nurses took care of me. They had access to every part of my body. They changed my condom catheter, emptied my bedpan, and saw me at my absolute worst. With the nurses, self-consciousness and vanity were forgotten luxuries. Unlike normal life, I couldn't hide behind a façade of nice clothing and role playing. My mind had adapted to the hospital situation without any conscious effort.

Chapter 6

Guillain Barré Syndrome

"If thou hast no name to be known by,
let us call thee devil. "
Othello, William Shakespeare

Dr. Singer stopped by to give me important information.

"John, we have the results of the spinal tap. The pressure, cell count, and protein content of the cerebrospinal fluid are all within normal limits. Your protein level is a little elevated, so we'll have to check it again, but we can now eliminate a number of previous possibilities. After a lengthy analysis, our diagnostic team believes your paralysis is due to an autoimmune disease called Guillain Barré Syndrome. We suspected it from the very first day. Would you like me to explain further?" This was the first definitive diagnosis I'd had since the paralysis began.

I blinked once.

"Well, it's a form of paralysis that comes on quickly. It was first described by a French doctor named Guillain Barré and it's sometimes referred to as French polio. The name merely describes a collection of symptoms and is descriptive rather than prescriptive. Its medical name is idiopathic polyneuritis, which in layman's terms means the inflammation of many nerves causing dysfunction. Each case is different and there is no specific treatment available. Your sensory nerves are working fine, but the covering of your motor nerves was attacked by your own immune system when it overreacted to the toxicity in your body. They will need time to regenerate the myelin sheath they lost. All of our tests and diagnostics indicate the cause is due to viral hepatitis. The prognosis for recovery is good."

Dr. Singer followed his explanation by adding, "I would like to do a second lumbar puncture now to get more up-to-date information and compare it with the results of the first. Are you okay with that?"

I blinked my agreement and he had a nurse witness my approval. Dr. Singer then rolled me on my side, gave me a local, and did another lumbar puncture. It was as well done as the first time. No problems and no pain. Some doctors naturally have the magic touch.

Now my paralysis had a name. I never heard of it before. I wondered how it was spelled. Based on Dr. Singer's pronunciation of "Ghee-yahn-bah-Ray" and the fact it was a French name, I figured it was spelled Guyon Beret, like the French hat. The diagnosis was certainly better than being told I had multiple sclerosis, Lou Gehrig's disease, or some other irreversible condition. Still, I didn't know much beyond that.

Dr. Singer had another item on his agenda. "John, I'm going to remove the IV and put in a nasogastric tube to get your nourishment directly into your stomach."

I was more than anxious to get rid of the painful IV needle in my arm that had to be changed so often.

Dr. Singer raised the head of my bed to put me in a sitting position. He unwrapped a Dobbhoff tube and lubricated the small mercury bulb on the end. He explained the bulb acted as a weight that helped pull the tube down my esophagus. Not being able to swallow, I couldn't help him. Slipping the bulb into my nose and maneuvering it past my pharynx, he continued feeding the tube in, inch by inch. Once the weighted bulb entered my esophagus, the tube moved more quickly.

"Okay, it's almost in. I want you to sit quietly and let gravity take it the rest of the way down into your stomach. I'll be back in about an hour to finish up." He left.

The NG tube in my nose was a new feeling. It felt different than the endotracheal tube I had in my nostril previously. It didn't hurt, but it didn't feel good either. I concentrated on relaxing while I watched television.

Dr. Singer returned as promised. He pushed the tube in a little farther until the mark on the tube showed it was in my stomach. To be sure it wasn't all tangled up somewhere en route, he put his stethoscope to my stomach and had a nurse push a little water through the tube while he listened for it to enter my stomach.

"I heard it. It's in your stomach," he said with a smile. Dr. Singer was an excellent doctor in spite of his youth.

Rosa came over and hooked me up to the new feeding system. This liquid stuff would undoubtedly keep me nourished, but I would have traded it in a New York minute for a chilidog with onions.

Not having eaten for a while, I daydreamed about real food. The thought of eating a chilidog became an ongoing obsession. There was something special about those fantastic flavors of meat, chili, and onions all mixed together.

I lay on my left side facing the dripfeed pump. I had something new to occupy my mind. I studied the directions on the side of the unit that told how to operate the pump, troubleshoot problems, and convert drops per minute into cc's. I studied everything in sight, including the number of soundproofing holes in the ceiling tiles and the design pattern on the drawcurtain by my bed.

I closed my eyes to rest and nodded off. A short time later, I felt someone's presence and opened my eyes. It was Hugh Whelpton, my friend from Western Industries. He must have slipped by the nurses because I had blinked "no" when the nurses asked me if I wanted any visitors besides Charlene and Chris. I really didn't want anyone seeing me in this condition. Hugh had known me when I was healthy and well groomed. What would he think of me now?

Hugh was his usual warm and friendly self. He said all the people at Western Industries sent their best wishes for my recovery and he brought me up to date on what was happening at the company. After a few minutes, I was glad my old friend had come to visit. It was nice to have a familiar face around.

Rosa came over and they talked about how I was doing. She briefed him on what the doctors had said about my condition. After a pleasant ten minutes listening to their conversation, Hugh said he had to leave but would return soon. I felt much better after his visit. My lousy appearance and sickly condition hadn't seemed to matter to him at all. He was truly a good friend.

A short while after Hugh left, a young woman in a staff coat came to the side of my bed and introduced herself.

"Hello Mr. Sueta. I'm Janis, a physical therapist. Dr. Singer has requested that you receive range-of-motion exercises every day to prevent contractures from forming in your joints. It's important to start doing ROM as soon as possible, before the contractures become irreversible."

It made sense, and yet I was being handled and jostled so much by the nurses all day that I really didn't want anyone else turning and twisting me. My body was extremely sensitive to handling. Any slight pressure on me was painful because my muscles had become flaccid and my nerve endings vulnerable. What I really wanted was to be left alone so I could rest. However, that was a foolish wish because I needed the constant care.

But, Janis was exactly the wrong type of physical therapist for me. She didn't have the light touch necessary for handling a patient in my weakened condition. Worse, she wasn't interested in what she was doing. As she bent my elbows and knees, her face was turned in the opposite direction, watching the television screen. The pain from her careless flexing was excruciating. I couldn't yell out, but I tried to let her know it was painful by moving my lower jaw from side to side. It was the only thing I could move to get her attention. She continued watching TV while she roughly bent and twisted my arms and legs.

At one point she turned her eyes in my direction and noticed my jaw moving.

She smiled and said, "Look, every time I bend your leg, your jaw moves." She thought that was cute, never realizing I was trying to tell her she was hurting me. Still smiling, she turned her attention back to the TV. After about 15 minutes of this torture, she was done and said, "I'll see you tomorrow."

I hoped not!

When a new shift came on duty, I never knew which nurse would be assigned to me. If it was one of my favorite nurses, I relaxed and felt a tremendous sense of relief because I knew for the next eight hours I would have good nursing care and be safe. It meant everything to me.

Of the twenty or so nurses and aides who worked on the ward's three shifts, seven were my favorites.They were a diverse group: male and female, black and white, American born, Asian, and Puerto Rican. In the group were four young women, Rosa, Linda, Anne, and Maureen, a young black male nurse named Gary, a fortyish male nursing aide named Norby, and the headnurse Theresa.

These nurses seemed to take a personal interest in me, though I didn't know why. I wasn't a special patient in any way. I couldn't talk, so they didn't know my personality except for my brief messages on the alphabet board. It obviously wasn't my physical self they liked because my appearance was a mess with matted hair, unshaven face, and a withered body with a lot of tubes stuck in it. I also required a lot of care. As far as I could see, there wasn't much about me to like.

Nevertheless, these young nurses made a connection with me. I saw it in their eyes, heard it in their voices, and felt it in their touch. They took excellent care of me and made me feel secure. Whenever one of them was assigned to me, I knew I'd be protected. They were the most important people in my life. They were my guardians around the clock.

I kept wondering why some nurses had made a personal connection with me. I had always believed that if I presented a nice physical appearance, was friendly, and had an impressive lifestyle, people would like and respect me. But, now I had none of those things.

Except for a sheet covering my body, I was physically naked. Psychologically, my inner self was as exposed as my body.

Years ago, I had written a college term-paper about the "inner self." My research showed me the inner self was a mixture of a person's inborn temperament and the culture which shaped it. We weren't born with a sense of self and had to learn who we were through interacting with the world around us. From the classic blending of nature-nurture, a self-image emerged and became "I." It was a person's most private self that harbored his deepest feelings and beliefs. It was who he consciously knew as "me."

I recalled making the analogy that the inner self was like the hub of a wagonwheel with the many roles a person played radiating outward from the central self like spokes. In the course of daily living, a person played the many roles of parent, spouse, friend, coworker, and others—but rarely revealed his true inner core, fearing exposure of his fears, insecurities, and imagined dark side. No one was what they appeared to be because they had adopted roles they believed were necessary to function socially.

Remembering all of this helped me to understand why nurses might bond with a patient like me. If nurses were able to see the true self of a patient who was in no position to play roles, they could relate to his basic humanity. It was ironical that seeing the inner self of a patient could be endearing rather than repellent. The very thing people tried so hard to hide from others was actually what touched others' deeper feelings. I thought of how foolish it was that people opened up their inner feelings and allowed their humanity to show through only when a traumatic event like sickness or tragedy stripped away their need to be guarded. It was during those traumatic times that people realized the inner selves they tried to hide weren't so terrible after all—that they were only human.

And so it was with me. Nurses must have related to the inner person they saw struggling for surival. In addition to their empathy for my plight, they could see glimpses of my inner self through the expressions of my eyes, my alphabet board communication, and through talking with Hugh and Charlene. Some began to know me in a personal way.

But, connecting with a patient's inner self could cause what I considered a "nurse's dilemma," wherein a nurse had to walk a fine line between maintaining her nursing objectivity or forming an emotional attachment. A patient's pitiful condition could make it difficult for her to stay emotionally detached. However, if she didn't keep her professional distance, she risked internalizing the patients' suffering. On the other hand, a nurse who kept a protective shell around her emotions might give care that was impersonal and minimal.

It seemed a common dilemma. A nurse who was attached to a patient was bound to feel hurt when a coveted patient left the hospital or didn't recover. It made her vulnerable. Paradoxically, it was when she dared to be more connected that she experienced the deepest fulfillment from the interaction. Allowing herself to be vulnerable was a two-edged sword that could be the source of her greatest pleasure or her deepest pain.

Hospice nurses dealt with the dilemma on a daily basis, but seemed to be able to cope because they had developed a mindset for dealing with terminal sickness and death. They balanced compassion with objectivity and kept a clear image of what their role was at all times. There seemed to be a switch in the mind that could be flipped to focus on the nursing task of easing the suffering rather than on the suffering itself.

The psychology of nurses fascinated me. I didn't know whether the high dropout rate of nurses I had read about proved not everyone had the temperament to be a nurse or whether better training would have helped them learn how to tolerate the many stresses. It was probably a combination of both.

After only a few weeks in the hospital, I became quite good at evaluating nurses. I could see that nurses were like any other profession: there were good ones and average ones— and even a few bad ones. Most patients could tell the difference. The good nurses had a distinctive way of doing things that was special. Injections were given with a minimum of discomfort because they were done unhurriedly and tenderly. Suctioning was performed carefully and patiently. Handling was gentle and the better nurses made sure you were comfortable before they moved on—they didn't flop you over, quickly jamb pillows behind your back, and walk away.

Good nurses cared about patients like me even when we were being difficult. They realized the frail persons inside the hospital gowns were completely different people in normal life. Suffering made us behave differently than we would have normally. Good nurses let us keep our dignity and showed us respect even when we didn't deserve it.

I wished one of my special nurses could be assigned to me permanently on each shift. Having primary nursing care instead of team nursing would have given me the peace of mind I badly needed.

I spelled out my wish on the alphabet board to Theresa, the headnurse whom I respected. She was a Philippina lady who was unbelievably kind. When Charlene and Chris or Hugh visited, she always came over to assure them I was being well cared for.

When I spelled out to Theresa that I'd like to have Rosa permanently assigned to me, she answered, "Mr. Sueta, we can't do that for many reasons. We don't want nurses to form personal relationships that might influence their nursing decisions. If Rosa was out sick or had the day off, the substitute wouldn't be familiar with your special needs. Furthermore, you require a lot of attention and one nurse would be overworked taking care of you every day. It just isn't possible Mr. Sueta, even if I wanted to."

I didn't completely agree because I felt it could be worked out in my case. My care could be shared by two or three of my favorite nurses. That would allow them to care for me on alternate days and have a fill-in when one wasn't on duty. I needed nurses who took an interest in me.

However, the headnurse prevailed. She was in charge of the ward and blinking my eyes at the alphabet board didn't give me much power to argue with her. Theresa was doing what she thought was best and I had to respect that.

I didn't win that one, but maybe I'd have better luck with my next request. I spelled out on the alphabet board to Dr. Singer that I wanted a different physical therapist. That request was granted because the next day a nice looking, middle-aged lady with a pleasant personality came.

"Good morning John. My name is Mary and I've been assigned as your physical therapist. I was told you have Guillain Barré Syndrome. I know something about it because I took care of an eighty year old man who had it. A friend of mine also had it. She's out of the hospital now and doing quite well. Her name is Jenny. If you'd like me to, I'll ask her to pay you a visit."

I blinked once.

As she began to gently give me range of motion, Mary explained, "What happened to you, John, is the myelin sheath, a fatty insulator that covers your motor nerves, was mistakenly attacked by your own immune system trying to fight a viral infection. The sheath was eaten away, causing inflammation and pressure on your motor nerves. Your neural messages were interrupted and your muscles became paralyzed without nerves to trigger them.

"When the virus is finally killed, the myelin cover will need time to regenerate. The regrowth will be proximo-distal, from the spinal chord outward to your fingers and toes, exactly in reverse of how it happened. It grows back very slowly, so you can see it takes a long time to grow from your spine to the tips of your toes. My eighty year old patient recovered after nine months." (She intentionally did not mention the 20% mortality rate from pneumonia or respiratory failure).

Mary finished my range of motion and said she would be back tomorrow.

I thought, "Nine months? That's an eternity. That's after Christmas. I can't wait that long. I'm a busy guy. I've got to get back to Western Industries and finish my projects. I have three houses that need to have mortgage payments made. Besides, the chief neurologist said I'd be out in thirty days. This thing came on in a few days so it should leave just as quickly. It will probably turn a sharp corner and I'll soon be back to normal. I'm not buying that nine months stuff."

The paralysis had happened like some bad sci-fi movie in which a giant hand had picked me up, put me in a strange place, and tied me down so I couldn't move, breathe, or speak. In an instant I was cut off from everything I had known. Every part of my former life was left in limbo. The paralysis had happened so hard and so fast, I didn't have time to adjust mentally.

At the time the paralysis struck, I was working long hours and earning a good salary, buying real estate and making other investments. My life had been filled with striving to make money. I had the typical illusion of what the so-called "good life" was all about. Owning an expensive car and a nice home, traveling, partying, eating in good restaurants, and wearing nice clothes were all part of the illusion. I believed those things were necessary for me to be happy. I had some of those things and wanted to get the rest. Once I had all this "stuff," I was sure I'd be happy.

Looking back, I saw that my former life was just like the ant farm I had bought for Chris when he was a boy. Through the glass front on the box, I watched the ants digging tunnels. They were constantly busy, carrying away grains of sand to make a new tunnel. However, the sand they carried out of a new tunnel was placed into an existing tunnel, filling it back up. They never stopped. They were instinctively driven to keep working despite the fact that they were endlessly repeating the same cycle of build, tear down, build, tear down, over and over. It made no sense. My life had also been an endless series of doing things to keep busy like the ants, never stopping to enjoy what I already had.

Here I was, paralyzed, on a ventilator fighting for my life, and money, possessions, and status meant nothing—absolutely nothing. I would have traded everything I owned for the ability to breathe on my own, walk, and eat real food. Those things truly mattered. It took a terrible illness to make me stop what I was doing and look at my life honestly. Otherwise, I would have continued following my false illusion of what was important.

I tried to picture what a truly good life would be like if I survived and left the hospital. I wouldn't need much money because I wouldn't want much, just a small car and enough money to get by on. I'd be happy to spend the rest of my life breathing fresh air, eating good meals, and enjoying the changing seasons. That's all I would ever want if I made it out of this hell. Anything more would just be frosting on the cake. An ordinary day would be a special day. A plain day would be a treasure.

It made sense. I remembered Henry Thoreau's criticism of false living in his classic book Walden, "The mass of men lead lives of quiet desperation, why should we live with such hurry and waste of life? Simplify, simplify."

If I ever got well, I wondered if I would follow Thoreau's wise advice or go back to my frantic pursuits like the ants neverending digging that lead nowhere?

My thoughts returned to the reality of my present condition. Mary's explanation of how long my recovery would take left me feeling depressed. Dr. Hanson had told me I'd be out in thirty days, but a part of me believed Mary might be right. The thought of being in the hospital for nine months, and possibly longer, was too much to accept at this time. I still wanted to believe in a sharp-corner recovery because I needed that belief to keep my hopes alive.

My positive thoughts were in daily conflict with my feelings of hopelessness. I had been in the hospital for weeks and saw no noticeable improvement. I had always believed that if I ever became seriously ill, my positive attitude would get me through it. I believed if I mentally willed myself to get better, it would happen. I believed in miracles.

I stared down at my lifeless hands. I concentrated as hard as I could and willed my numbed fingers to move. I mentally commanded them, "Move! Move! I feel the life force surging through you. Move! I feel you moving. Move!"

I stayed focused as I repeated those positive affirmations over and over, watching and waiting for a slight twitch. There was no response. I kept repeating the affirmations. There was still no movement.

After many attempts, I began to lose hope, but I still wasn't convinced that my mind couldn't force my hands to move, even if it was only a twitch. I wasn't someone who gave up easily. I tried to channel every ounce of energy into my fingers. I used every bit of willpower and determination I could muster as I repeated, "Move. I know you can move. I feel you moving. Move!"

Countless repetitions later, I knew it wasn't going to happen. There wasn't the slightest hint of movement. I continued trying until I became mentally exhausted and closed my eyes in despair. This wasn't the make-believe world of Hollywood miracles, this was real life.

My old belief that I could fight off any disease by sheer willpower was fading, but not gone. Many times afterward I focused all my energy on my hands and feet and willed them to move. I concentrated with every fiber of my being and failed every time. The immense effort always left me feeling exhausted and depressed.

I had been in the hospital for over a month. My condition was no better. I could only blink my eyes, move my lower jaw, and control my eliminations. My once firm muscles were becoming mushy and useless. The toxins were still waging war with my white blood corpuscles. In the battle, my liver had become inflamed and caused daily fevers.

My wretched situation seemed so hopeless that I couldn't help thinking of ways to end it. Irrational ideas of suicide paraded before my mind. How would I do it? Pills? Carbon monoxide?

I pictured myself swallowing a bunch of pills—but I didn't have any pills and I couldn't swallow them if I had them. So, I pictured myself sitting in my car in a closed garage with the engine running, but I was in a hospital bed totally paralyzed. Neither of those ideas made any sense.

I wondered, "If I had a control button on the bed that would end my life, would I push it? Would I give up the possibility of getting well?" I had to mentally laugh at the irony of it. With my inability to move my fingers, I couldn't push a button.

I considered asking to be disconnected from the ventilator, but I knew the hospital would never allow it.

All those ideas were impossibly ridiculous. They were simply my analytical mind considering every conceivable alternative. I knew I'd never have taken any of those ways out, but it was depressing to be so helpless that I couldn't even consider them.

When Rosa came over to talk to me, I closed my eyes. I was too depressed to talk to anyone. She sensed something was wrong.

"What's the matter John? Here's the board. Open your eyes and spell it out. C'mon John, open your eyes and talk to me."

I kept them closed. She kept trying. I kept ignoring her.

Finally, she put down the alphabet board and gave me a lesson I would remember for the rest of my time in the hospital.

"John, don't make the nurses think you've lost your spirit and given up. They'll lose interest in you. People reflect back to you the same feelings you show them. If you don't care, they won't care. So snap out of it."

That bit of wisdom hit home. It was all right to be depressed, but I'd better not show it to those I depended on for critical support. As close as Rosa and I were, I knew she would not put up with any self-pitying nonsense. In any relationship, if you cross a certain line, you jeopardize the relationship. I opened my eyes and blinked once for "okay."

I was learning how to survive in a hospital....

Chapter 7

The Power of "No"

"Power, alas! naught but misery brings!"
Thomas Haynes Bayly (1797-1839)

There were three TVs in the ward. One hung on the wall directly in front of me. The remote control was on the pillow next to my head, but I couldn't push the buttons so it stayed on the same channel all day. I saw every repeat of The Twilight Zone, Bonanza, and MASH over and over until I knew every episode by heart.

One day the TV's remote control was left on my pillow, halfway under my right ear. I unconsciously rolled my head to move away from it. Then the reality of my movement struck me. I had rolled my head!

I couldn't believe it. It was the first time a major movement had occurred. I was ecstatic! As I rolled my head back and forth, my cheek hit the TV remote button and flipped the channels. It felt wonderful. I was actually controlling something outside myself. This was my first important physical interaction with my environment since I entered the hospital. After months of total helplessness, I was physically causing something to happen. I felt a tremendous power. I now realized how important it was to have control over something in my external world.

I pressed the remote button over and over with my cheek, flipping channels, until the remote slid down the pillow and out of my reach.

"Damn, I wasn't through yet," I thought to myself. I had lost my source of control. But, more important than just being able to change the channels, I had a new power. By rolling my head back and forth, I could now shake my head to say "No."

When the afternoon nurse began to turn me on my side, I used my newly found power and shook my head "No." I was much more comfortable lying on my back and I was tired of constantly being placed on my side. The nurse didn't stop, so I kept shaking my head "No" until she did. I had intimidated her and she gave in to me.

She never should have let me do that because I laid on my back for the whole shift and part of the night shift. It felt good, but I paid a price. The skin on my buttock formed a red rash, the first sign of a bedsore.

Lying too long in one position could also cause lung problems. I had been in the hospital for almost two months and my lungs consistently had fluid in them that required constant suctioning. What was causing my ongoing pneumonia? Were fluids forming in my lungs from lying too long in one position?

Whatever the cause, it was a serious problem. I needed suctioning every hour, more frequently on some days. Rosa and most other nurses did it dutifully without a fuss, but others became tired of the repetitive labor and ignored me until they believed suctioning was absolutely necessary. They waited until my breathing made the telltale rale sounds or they noticed dyspnea. One disgruntled nurse wrote in her report, "Patient wants constant suctioning and very little mucus found." Her comment echoed what many nurses felt.

Nurses knew that a mass of thick fluids in my airways would restrict ventilator oxygen from passing into my lungs. However, what many nurses didn't know was that even a small glob of the thick, sticky mucus could adhere to the walls of my trachea or bronchial tubes and form a partial membrane across the opening. With the ventilator set to deliver the bare minimum of oxygen, even a small restriction was a problem. I needed every bit of oxygen I could get. I knew immediately when I wasn't receiving enough oxygen because I felt my face flush as my temperature rose from hypoxia.

In normal life, whenever I got a small bit of saliva or phlegm caught in my throat, I automatically coughed and cleared my airways without even realizing I had done so. But now, I couldn't cough and needed suctioning to clear the slightest blockage. I remembered that President Reagan had been given the Heimlich maneuver when he was choking on one small peanut. Unless a nurse personally experienced breathing on a ventilator, she couldn't possibly realize the effects of even a small obstruction.

When a nurse did respond to my signals and suctioned me, the vacuum broke the webbed blockage. However, when she saw only a small amount of "harmless" mucus in the vacuum tube, she believed I had overreacted and the suctioning was a waste of her time. This happened time after time, so a few nurses believed I was too demanding and was "manipulating" them for attention. That was their reality. They had no way of knowing the truth unless they had been taught the subtleties of respiratory distress.

When one of the more skilled nurses suctioned me, I received wonderful bursts of oxygen pumped into me from the AMBU bag used between insertions of the catheter. It offered me temporary relief from the constant struggle with the ventilator. My whole body responded with a blessed "Aaahh." It wasn't the reason I wanted suctioning because most nurses used the AMBU bag sparingly and I received less oxygen than I would have from the ventilator, but it was a pleasant relief when done by the right nurse.

Whenever my anxiety level became intense, I tried to relieve the stress by recalling jokes I enjoyed in the past. Humor helped to ease the tension. The vacuum tube's sucking sound reminded me of the joke about a guy at a party who kept eating peanuts till he emptied the bowl. When he apologized to the elderly hostess, the old lady said, "It's okay sonny, I already sucked all the chocolate off them." Thinking of that joke always made me chuckle inside and relieved some of my stress.

Chest X-rays confirmed my ongoing pneumonia. Dr. Singer percussed my chest and auscultated my lungs, trying to determine its severity. Until now, he had taken no direct action. He theorized the pneumonia might be caused by cardiovascular disease, an infection, kidney disease, or pleurisy.

"John, you can't seem to lose that fluid on your lungs, so I'd like to do a thoracentesis. It isn't a complicated procedure. I'll draw some fluid from your lungs and I hope it will tell us more about the problem."

I was turned onto my side. He didn't have to tell me not to move or cough because I couldn't anyway. The long needle puncture was totally painless and it was over in a few minutes.

"I'll send this to the lab and let you know if we find anything."

After the procedure, the nurses let me rest for a few hours before turning me. When they turned me, nurses usually wedged pillows under my back and between my legs before they placed the pillow under my head. They were so intent on not letting me roll onto my back that they allowed my head to dangle downward on my limp neck while they arranged the other pillows. I could never understand why so many nurses fixed my head pillow last when it should have been done first.

Sometimes when a nurse turned me on my side, I felt a dizzying rush that caused me to almost pass out. The dizziness only happened when I was turned onto my right side. I didn't know why.

With few exceptions, I was turned every two or three hours. I was receiving excellent care, but the constant handling and sleep interruptions were wearing me out. The only semblance of comfort I had was when the nurses left me on my back, which they seldom did. Instead of getting two hours of comfort on my back, they kept turning me from one side to the other because their training must have taught them to keep a patient off his back. No sooner had one shift of nurses finished, then a fresh, new shift took up where the other shift left off.

In my weakened state, I disliked the constant handling. However, the nurses wanted to prevent the already reddened area on my buttock from turning into a decubitus. If allowed to lie too long on my back, the bony projections in my shoulders and buttocks could press on my flesh and create wet spots which could then turn into open, ulcerated sores that were susceptible to infection--like the one that killed Christopher Reeve.

Despite that danger, I sometimes tried to communicate with Rosa and the other nurses that I didn't want to be turned so often, but they did what they thought best. At the time it upset me, but later I recognized it was good nursing because it would have been much easier for them not to bother.

I thought, "Happiness is a day without being touched." I pictured what it would be like to be left alone for one whole day. How wonderful it would be to live in an apartment all by myself with no one to touch me all day long. It was an irrational fantasy because I needed turning, suctioning, foodbag changes, and all the other care.

To avoid being turned, I'd sometimes "play possum" by pretending I was asleep. If a nurse believed I was getting some valuable sleep, she might leave me alone. It also depended on whether she wanted to get her duties out of the way or whether she was willing to postpone them. Many patients used this pretense to avoid being turned, getting shots, or having blood drawn. However, most nurses were aware of the possum game and told them, "I know you're not asleep. Let's get this over with."

An hour later, Charlene and Chris arrived. They didn't visit often because it was a long drive and coming to see me lying there with sick and dying men all around me was too disturbing. I understood. They did manage to come once a week to bring news from the outside. Rosa taught them how to use the alphabet board and that helped lighten their visits.

Charlene tried hard to cheer me up by using humor, just as I tried to do. In that hectic environment, it wasn't easy. My inability to talk reminded Charlene of a joke she thought might brighten my spirits.

She began, "This old man was walking in the woods when a frog appeared in his path. The frog spoke in a sweet, feminine voice saying, 'Old man, if you pick me up and kiss me, I'll turn into a beautiful princess and grant you your every desire.'

"The old man picked up the frog and put it in his pocket.

"In a short while, the sweet voice came from his pocket repeating, 'Old man, I said if you kiss me, I will turn into a princess who will grant you your every desire.'

"The old man angrily replied, 'I heard you. I heard you. But at my age, I'd rather have a talking frog.' "

I couldn't physically smile, but I smiled within. Keeping a sense of humor was important.

An hour after they left, Rosa said I had a lady visitor named Jenny and asked if I wanted to see her. It was my physical therapist's friend. I had left instructions that I didn't want any visitors except Charlene and Chris unless the nurses checked with me first. I may have lost my vanity with the staff, but I sure didn't want anyone else seeing me like this. I needed a shave and a haircut. Besides all the tubes sticking out of me, my emaciated body had a bloated stomach that looked like I had swallowed a watermelon, with liquid sloshing around inside whenever I was turned. It surprised me how fast muscles I had spent years developing had turned soft and weak in such a short time.

Since Jenny was a stranger and didn't know how I looked before, I didn't feel the same embarrassment. I blinked once to agree I'd see her. My physical therapist had said Jenny had had Guillain Barré too, so I felt she might have more information about my disease.

Jenny came to my bedside. "Hi John. I'm Jenny. Mary said she told you about me."

I blinked once.

Jenny was an attractive woman about my age.

"I had Guillain Barré too. Mine wasn't quite as bad as yours, but I was on a ventilator and I couldn't walk for months. My joints were really painful."

She didn't use the alphabet board, so I could only listen. Jenny proceeded to describe her experience in detail. Afterward she said, "I was fed through a tube like you and my husband asked me what I wanted to eat as soon as I could swallow. The very first thing that came to my mind was a chilidog with lots of onions."

I wanted to say, "Me too! Me too! That's what I want."

Jenny continued, "As soon as I got rid of that darn NG tube, he brought me a chilidog. I savored every mouthful. What a joy it was to be eating again. You'll be eating real food soon, John."

She continued, "One day, my feet began twitching all of a sudden. It startled me. I kept wiggling my toes till I got tired. With physical therapy, it only took a few weeks before I was starting to walk. And here I am. I still get tired and can't walk great distances, but I'm improving every day."

She was confirming my belief that my paralysis would also turn around and leave as quickly as it came.

"What a shame," she sympathized as she saw my badly discolored arms where countless syringe sticks had turned them black and blue.

She smiled and wished me good luck as she left. She was a wonderful lady who had taken the time to visit a complete stranger in order to offer encouragement and hope. I appreciated it and wished I could have thanked her with more than just my eyes.

After she left, I thought about what she said about wanting a chilidog. Her too. I wondered what the heck it was about a chilidog that people craved when they hadn't tasted food for a while?

Chapter 8

Rational and Irrational Fears

"The only thing we have to fear is fear itself."
President Franklin D. Roosevelt

On morning rounds, a team of doctors stood at the foot of my bed and discussed my case. Usually they spoke as if I wasn't even there, but today they spoke softly so I couldn't hear what they were saying. I could tell they were talking about me because they looked over at me from time to time. I figured if they didn't want me to hear, it must be bad. That made me nervous. I became even more nervous when Dr. Marshall, the respiratory doctor, and his assistant went over to the ventilator's control panel.

The panel was too high for me to see what they were doing, but from their body movements, I could tell they were making adjustments.

"Leave it alone! Don't turn it down," my mind kept thinking over and over—but I knew they would make adjustments. They were either going to reset the oxygen level or number of breaths.

I was on 14 breaths a minute with 23% oxygen. They turned it down to 12 breaths. I noticed the awful difference immediately because my efforts to breathe were no longer in harmony with the machine. Whenever they made any change, I knew I had to begin a new fight against oxygen deprivation. I was tired of the whole damned struggle. I was unaware that I was on Ritalin to alleviate my anxiety.

The respiratory staff wrote in my records that I was "too preoccupied with the ventilator" and they didn't want to cause me further anxiety, so they kept every phase of the weaning process a secret. I had no idea that they were gradually weaning me off the machine by decreasing the percentage of oxygen and number of breaths per minute. I thought they were just adjusting the settings back and forth according to my condition at the time. All I knew was each change left me struggling harder to breathe.

Probably very old or very sick patients who were not being weaned were receiving generous amounts of ventilator oxygen, but for someone like me on a weaning schedule, the amount of air was constantly kept at a level that forced me to try to breath on my own.

I kept looking for meaningful signs that I was improving. Without their feedback, I didn't know that, at times, I could now breathe strongly enough to trigger the machine into giving me up to four extra breaths a minute. The fact that I was able to assist the machine showed a marked improvement that I wasn't even aware of. If I hadn't been in a constant state of anxiety, I might have realized that Dr. Marshall's ventilator adjustments were not made without good reason and were actually signs my breathing had improved. But, the thought never entered my mind because I didn't see the big picture and was focusing all my energy on my immediate efforts to breathe. I felt so short of oxygen all the time that I didn't see the reduction in ventilator output as something positive.

If the weaning process had been fully explained to me, it would have eliminated much of my dread. Had I been included as a partner in the process, my improvements, however slight, would have inspired me and I would have formed a better mindset to deal with the breathing adjustments I was forced to make.

Unfortunately, I remained ignorant of the weaning process and all my thoughts were on adjusting to each new ventilator setting. After the change, I told myself, "Inhale, two, three, four, inhale, two, three, four, inhale...." On the first count I inhaled, on counts two, three, and four, I slowly exhaled.

It was mentally grueling, but after about an hour, I had the new timing down, "Inhale, two, three, four, inhale. Beautiful. Two, three, four, inhale." Once I had the rhythm going well, I focused on getting the sigh. "Inhale, two, three, four, inhale. Damn, a little too soon...inhale, two, three, four, inhale. Got it—aaah."

I counted all day long, minute after minute, hour after hour. I counted while watching TV. I even counted while using the alphabet board. The "inhale-two-three-four-inhale" rhythm was always in the background of my thinking. I believed I had to get every bit of oxygen I could in order to survive.

After the last change, I thought that if I dozed off, I would stop counting and miss getting full breaths. If that happened, would I pass out from hypoxia? Would I suffocate to death? I couldn't take a chance. I didn't allow myself to sleep even when they dimmed the lights at ten o'clock. I forced myself to stay awake and kept counting. In a sleepless daze, I counted all through the night and the next day. I had to stay awake. I had to count!

Whenever I dozed off for a few seconds, I quickly snapped awake. My first thought was, "Am I breathing? Count."

During the second night, I couldn't continue the battle to stay awake. I was completely exhausted and, despite all my efforts, I fell soundly asleep.

I shouldn't have worried. Mother Nature came to my rescue. During sleep, my autonomic nervous system took over my breathing rhythm and slowed my heartrate to a comfortable beat. I needed less oxygen and my ventilator had a guarantor that pumped the set number of breaths even when I stopped assisting. Mother Nature and the ventilator did their jobs and I got some much needed rest.

When I awoke, I realized it was safe for me to sleep, but I still counted while I was awake to make sure I'd catch the full volume and the sigh.

During all the hours of breathing difficulties, my special nurses made life bearable. Anne and Gary were two of my "special seven."

Anne was an attractive brunette in her mid-twenties. She was a true nurse who did total patient care. Some nurses only did the required duties, but Anne did more. Whenever she was assigned to me, she made sure I had regular bowel movements despite the extra cleanup work involved. Back rubs were never omitted. Before she turned me, she gave my arms and legs light range of motion. For my hygiene, Anne shampooed my hair and brushed my teeth. Everything was done with a pleasant attitude.

I heard Dr. Singer ask the headnurse what Anne's name was because he recognized her skills and wanted to know who she was. Competent nurses stood out from the crowd.

Gary was a young, thin, muscular black fellow whose nursing ability was only matched by his compassion and patience. He never showed the slightest annoyance in having to suction me, no matter how often it had to be done. He did it by the book, cleanly, carefully, and thoroughly. When he finished, my lungs and trachea felt clear and my lungs were rested from getting the proper amount of oxygen during bagging.

After he turned me, he always looked into my eyes while he replaced the pillows to make sure I was comfortable. If I blinked twice, he kept adjusting the pillows until I blinked once. Sometimes it took many adjustments, but he didn't mind.

Gary regularly communicated with me using the alphabet board, so he knew exactly how I was feeling and what I needed. Once, while we were using the alphabet board, I spelled out "please" before I asked him to do something because I felt guilty about asking him for so much help.

He interrupted my spelling and said, "John, it's really not necessary to waste your energy saying 'please.' It's no bother. Just tell me what you want and I'll do it." How do you measure the value of a nurse like that?

However, the secure feelings I got from my special nurses didn't eliminate the unending stress of struggling to breathe and to move. The long struggle was gradually wearing me down.

All the normal ways of relieving stress were not available to me. I couldn't actively deal with the stress. I had no way to burn off the built-up tension through physical activity. Frustration and tension were bottled up inside me with no outlet for expression. In my increasingly exhausted condition, it was becoming harder and harder to deal with the stress.

Life in the intensive care unit was wretched. I watched a dozen men die in the beds next to me. Some went quietly, others groaned in agony with every breath till their last. Lying paralyzed and without a voice, the world around me was a frightening place. Anxiety was my constant companion.

Some of my fears were real—and the ones that were only in my mind, felt just as real. Real and imagined fears were all tangled together. I became anxious when any stranger came near my bed. What did he want? What was he going to do? In my vulnerable condition, any stranger was an imagined threat. I was wary of everyone except the staff I knew well and trusted. Mostly, I dreaded when anyone went near the ventilator control panel.

When a new shift came on duty, I was afraid of being assigned the wrong nurse. When the ventilator tubes needed changing, I was afraid an unskilled respiratory therapist would keep me disconnected too long. I dreaded blood-drawing from staff who stuck me too many times.

Checking my heartrate on the digital readout above me showed my heart was beating at a high rate. How long could my overworked heart keep pumping at that pace? Would it soon give out? One night the heart monitor alarm sounded, but a bedside EKG had the normal three peak pattern, showing it was simply the result of my anxiety.

I dreaded every X-ray. The beeping sound of the portable X-ray machine coming down the hall was frightening. It meant my limp body was going to be propped up for a chest X-ray with my unsupported head flopping around as they jammed a cold, hard film plate behind my back.

I worried about overexposure to the radiation. Throughout my life, I had limited the number of X-rays I allowed, even from the dentist. Now I was continually getting X-rayed and I had no way of stopping it. The technician told me not to worry because the amount of radiation was not significant, but I noticed the staff hurried out of the room till the X-rays were finished.

The thought of a fire or an earthquake was upsetting because I knew, in a triage situation, bedridden patients were the last to be evacuated and in an extreme emergency were left behind. One night, I felt a large earthquake tremor and the electrical power went off, leaving the ward in darkness and my ventilator stopped. I nervously waited till the emergency generators kicked in.

Loud noises were especially frightening and my nerves jumped every time I heard one. My instinctive reaction sent adrenalin racing through my body. Without the ability to either fight or take flight, even small noises that a normal person wouldn't notice became magnified and penetrated to the bone.

Most housekeepers didn't use common sense when they mopped around the beds. They regularly bumped the bed with their brooms and mops, causing nerve-wracking vibrations and noise. They carelessly let the handle on the mop-wringing pail snap back with a loud, metallic clanging. After emptying wastebaskets, they dropped them back down on the floor instead of carefully placing them down. I hated to think of how those loud sounds affected comatose patients.

Staff members didn't realize the distress they caused when they dropped something that clattered or when they made other unnecessary noises. One day, a nursing aide stood by my bed chewing peanuts, unaware of the effect the grinding noise had on me. Each crunch sent shivers down my spine.

In past years, I remembered how hospital staffs talked softly around patients, but now they sometimes hollered to one another across the room. I had no right to expect a churchlike quiet, but I did expect more common sense. One day they would all be patients too and then they would understand.

I knew that no nurse could truly understand my fears. To fully comprehend my inner world, a nurse would have to imagine the frustration of lying in bed with every part of her body tightly strapped down so she couldn't move a single muscle. To understand what it was like breathing on a ventilator, she would have to imagine a wet towel covering her nose and mouth and the more she tried to breathe, the tighter the towel stuck to her face. No matter how hard she struggled to breathe, she could only suck in just enough air to stay alive. While totally unable to move and feeling in constant danger of suffocating, she would then have to imagine having painful blood drawings, daily fevers, and ongoing pneumonia. Finally, she would have to imagine her mouth taped shut, so she couldn't express her feelings of utter frustration from losing total control of her life.

Some nurses were more perceptive and insightful, and therefore more understanding than others, but none could fully understand my reality.

Chapter 9

The Only Thing Constant Is Change

"There is in the worst of fortune the best
of chances for a happy change."
Euripides (485 B.C.)

When Dr. Singer stopped by on his morning rounds, he told me he was being rotated to a different ward and I'd be getting a new doctor. I wished I could have told him how much I valued his excellent care. He would be a fine doctor when he finished his training. I tried to say it all with my eyes.

He smiled and waved goodbye as he walked away.

Later that morning, his replacement came by to introduce himself.

"Good morning John. I'm Dr. Sochat. Do you remember me? I was in the ER the night you were admitted."

I blinked twice. I didn't remember any of the people from that night. I was in too much distress.

I felt an immediate connection with this friendly young doctor in training and I was relieved my new doctor was someone I had a rapport with.

Dr. Sochat gave my vital signs a thorough check and said he would see me later that afternoon. After he left, I was visited by different doctors throughout the day, both in groups and individually. I thought they were all somehow involved in my case and I was impressed that I was the focus of so much attention. But my bubble was burst when Rosa told me they were medical students and interns who were only coming to observe my unusual disease as part of their education in this training hospital.

That afternoon, Dr. Sochat returned. He rechecked my lungs by percussing and auscultating.

"I've read your charts and see that you've had ongoing fluid on your lungs. We've been suctioning you often and we've used the heavy vibrator to loosen up the congestion, but I still hear the fluid, especially in your right lung. The thoracentesis didn't tell us anything except that you seem to be effusing fluids into your lungs."

I was aware that being immobile over a long period of time could lead to many health problems including pneumonia, but where was the fluid coming from?

"John, I'd like to schedule you for a bronchoscopy. It's a non-invasive operation where an ENT doctor inserts a tube into your bronchial tubes and suctions out the fluids. The tube has a lens on the end of it so he can see through an eyepiece exactly what he's doing. It's a much more precise way of clearing your lungs and at the same time see what's going on down there."

I was for anything that might help rid me of the fevers and constant suctioning. I gave my consenting eye blink to him and the witnessing nurse.

A few hours after Dr. Sochat left, an unfamiliar doctor arrived. "Mr. Sueta, I'm Dr. Chen from the ENT Department. I was told by Dr. Sochat that he explained the procedure to you, so I don't see any reason not to get started. If at any time you feel any discomfort, just blink your eyes."

The nurse cranked the head of my bed up so I was in a sitting position. Dr. Chen took a bronchoscope out of his medical bag and inserted the catheter down my trachea and into one of my bronchial tubes. The inserted end of the suction tube had a lighted lens on it. The top end he held in his hand had a suction pump with two eyepiece connections through which he and another observer could watch the procedure.

I felt no discomfort at all as he moved the catheter around and vacuumed out the fluid. While he worked, different nurses peeked into the second eyepiece of the bronchoscope to observe. At one point, he had a nurse hold the extra eyepiece to my eye so I could watch too. It was fascinating to see inside my lungs. Within fifteen minutes, the procedure was finished. I had felt absolutely no discomfort and actually enjoyed the whole thing. Dr. Chen was superbly skilled; he had "the touch."

Later that afternoon, a young woman came to give me range of motion. Mary, my physical therapist for the past weeks, was not available and this therapist was filling in. She was a young woman who gave me the impression she was new at the job. She didn't quite know how far to bend my limbs, but that was better than overdoing it. When she rolled me onto my right side, I felt the same dizzying rush in my head that I had sometimes experienced in the past. I assumed the dizziness was caused by being rolled onto my side. But why did it only happen when I was turned onto my right side? I had to give that some thought.

The young therapist finished my ROM and rolled me on my back before she left.

About once a week, one of the older Filippina nurses had the other nurses help her get me into the cardiac chair. It was folded down flat and wheeled next to my bed. After a pullsheet was slipped under me, they slid me onto the flattened chair.

The transfer never went smoothly. Any part of my body that flopped loosely without someone supporting it was often twisted and sprained—most often my neck. Once in the chair, the back support was raised to put me in a sitting position and I was strapped in tightly.

It felt good to be sitting up, looking around the ward from an upright position. Lying in bed for so many weeks and looking up at people was unnatural. I wanted to sit up and see things in a normal way and not feel like a helpless patient lying flat on my back.

Unfortunately, after about ten minutes, the nice feeling turned into discomfort. I couldn't shift my weight around like people do automatically after they have been sitting in one position too long. First I felt pressure on my buttocks. The pressure gradually increased until it became a prickly pain. After another ten minutes it felt like I was sitting on a thousand tiny needles. I couldn't shift my position even the fraction of an inch it took to relieve the unbearable stinging.

Some days I was able to sit for a torturous hour. I didn't know the nurses had orders to keep me in the chair as long as possible. I thought they just didn't want to put me back in bed so soon after expending so much effort to get me into the chair. It felt wonderful when they finally put me back in bed.

After dozing off, I was wakened by my friend Hugh.

"Hi, John. I brought you a little something." He opened his attaché case and pulled out a metal bracket and attached it to the bed's headboard. Then he pulled out a cardboard chart with writing on it and clamped it to the bracket.

"John, I know you were studying Spanish before, so I made something for you to work on."

Hugh adjusted the chart to about twelve inches from my eyes. On it, he'd carefully handprinted some Spanish vocabulary and grammar.

Now I could do something worthwhile during the day instead of just watching television. The nurses could swing the bracket with the card out of their way when caring for me and then swing it back when they were done. It was an exceptionally thoughtful thing for Hugh to have done. My special nurses made sure the chart was always in position for me to study.

That Spanish chart served another purpose—a much more important purpose. To staff who didn't know me well, I might be seen as just another half-conscious, mindless patient. The Spanish chart showed nurses, doctors, and other personnel that there was a thinking human being inside the inert body. Seeing the chart, they understood a real person was inside who was capable of rational thought. That realization changed the relationships for the better between some staff members and me.

Rosa was assigned to me for the day. It could have been coincidence, but I noticed that my favorite nurses were assigned to me most of the time. Then it dawned on me that it was more than just coincidence. Theresa, the headnurse, was assigning me my favorite nurses as often as she could while still maintaining a balance of other nurses. She was a great headnurse.

The ward bustled with morning activity. A new patient was brought in to the bed next to me. He must have been in great pain because he yelled loudly, hour after hour. I didn't know his physical problem, but he disturbed the whole ward with his groaning and yelling.

As the nurses tended to my new neighbor, I heard them call him Murphy. When Rosa stopped by, I spelled out on the board, "Who?" and turned my head in Murphy's direction.

"Same as you, John. The doctors think he has Guillain Barré. The reason he's yelling so much is because he's scared. He may have some pain, but mostly it's his fear of the paralysis that is still progressing. You know what he's going through better than I do."

I blinked once.

Murphy was about sixty years old, but he looked eighty. He was a tall, rawboned guy. Soon, Murphy began having visitors. They came and they came and they came, all day and evening. I could not believe the enormous number of visitors he had. There must have been fifty people who visited him that day. They were young and old, of all nationalities, in all manner of dress. I wondered who this guy was to have so many visitors. Were they family or friends? Was he a minister, a celebrity, or what? They brought flowers, held his hand, and consoled him. They had a calming effect on him and he was more quiet while they were there. The procession of visitors came every day.

Two of Murphy's visitors sometimes stopped by my bed to say hello and cheer me up. I appreciated their thoughtfulness. One was a pretty, redheaded woman named Virginia, and the other a jovial young man named Bill.

Rosa showed Virginia how to use the alphabet board, so one day I asked Virginia, "Who you?"

She candidly replied, "We're from Alcoholics Anonymous. Murphy is one of us."

The support the members of AA were giving Murphy was wonderful and I admired their togetherness. I had always respected the work of their organization and now I respected them even more.

The next day, Murphy's paralysis affected his breathing and he was taken to surgery for a tracheotomy and placed on a ventilator. That ended his yelling. He stayed on the ward for two weeks before they transferred him to the rehabilitation ward. I didn't know it, but Murphy and I would be seeing each other many times in the future.

I was expecting a visit from Charlene and Chris at around eight o'clock. I looked at the clock. Two more hours. My usual late afternoon fever was burning up my body. I could feel its heat on my face and the nausea starting. I hoped the fever would be gone before Charlene and Chris arrived because during their last visit, nurses had to put cold washrags on my forehead to cool me down. I had pretended I was all right, but

71

they left so the nurses could take care of my fever.

Charlene and Chris arrived at eight o'clock. My fever had gone down enough to allow me to focus on the unsettling information Charlene told me.

"John, I hate to bother you now, but I'm taking care of your mail and you have a lot of overdue bills. Your mortgage payments are all overdue and you're getting letters of foreclosure. I don't know what to do."

She picked up the board and I spelled, "Sell Dahlia house."

The house on Dahlia Street in Imperial Beach had enough equity in it to make the other two payments for a while. I hated to sell it because it was near the ocean and my dream was to build condominiums on the land. Now I had no choice. I needed the money.

Charlene left and I knew my favorite piece of property would soon be gone. I felt bad about having to sell the property I loved so dearly and I cursed my helplessness to do anything about it. The longer I stayed in the hospital, the more my outside world was crumbling. It was difficult to deal with the feeling of being so completely powerless to preserve the things I had worked so hard for.

At that point, I thought things were bad, but they got worse. One of the night nurses disliked me intensely and her nursing reflected her animosity. She saw me as a hopelessly ill patient whose constant care was a nuisance. I had previously complained about her poor nursing care to the night doctor, but nothing was done. The alphabet board was inadequate to fully express my thoughts and the doctor probably thought I was overreacting.

During the night, my mucus was flowing badly and I needed frequent suctioning, but the night nurse suctioned me only when *she* decided I needed it and scolded me repeatedly for bothering her.

At one point, when I signaled that I needed suctioning, she came over and said harshly, "I'm not going to suction you. I did it only an hour ago, so don't blink your eyes or shake your head cause I'm not going to suction you till I'm good and ready."

She proceeded to ignore me even though she could tell by my labored breathing and gurgling sounds that my airways needed suctioning badly. I felt I was going to choke as I fought to inhale as much air as I could from the ventilator.

Despite the frightening situation, I knew I had to be very careful about making an enemy of her. Alone, at night on a darkened, quiet ward was no place to arouse a nurse's anger. There were dozens of ways an irate nurse could retaliate against a patient she intensely disliked.

After what seemed like an hour, she finally decided it was time. She was angry and suctioned me crudely. During the suctioning, she vented her anger and whispered, "You just lie there and don't want to get well. I'm sick and tired of you. I'd like to shut you up for good."

I was shaken!! Without being able to move my arms in defense and no voice to yell, I was completely at her mercy. Had she really meant it or was she just venting her anger? I couldn't take a chance. It was enough warning for me not to bother her again. The next time I needed suctioning, I'd try to get the attention of the other night nurse on duty.

I decided not to tell anyone what she had said because I didn't want to say anything that might create a worse situation. When I had previously complained about her, nothing had been done. No one would believe me anyway. How much credibility would I have by spelling out my claim on an alphabet board in tedious, one letter at a time sentences?

Nurses like her probably entered the field for the wrong reasons and did only what was minimally necessary to keep their jobs. They kept themselves emotionally distant from patients, put in their eight hours, and went home.

Mercifully, morning came and the day shift nurses began arriving. Their hair and clothing were wet and I could hear them telling the night shift that it was pouring rain outside.

Rain... it sounded wonderful to me. It was springtime, but in intensive care, every day was the same. There were no seasons, no weather changes. The environment inside completely controlled. The temperature was always the same and the recirculated air was stale and didn't have the fragrant smell of fresh air. The windows were behind my head so I never saw the sun or sky. My visual world was the television on the wall and the hospital staff at the nurses' station across the aisle. My only contact with the outside world was the bright warmth of the sun on my head when the drapes were opened.

Today, it was raining. The nurses coming on duty were trying to dry off and were complaining to the night nurses who would soon be going out into the downpour. I remembered how I used to hate rain too. Soaked clothing, wet hair, and traffic jams had been nuisances in the past.

But, now it was different. Lying there in the intensive care unit, I actually envied the nurses who had gotten wet. I thought, "How wonderful a cool raindrop would feel on my face. Don't they realize what a luxury it is to be able to walk outside, breathe fresh air, and feel the cool, refreshing rain on their faces? If I ever get outside and it's raining, I'm going to enjoy every minute of it. I'm going to turn my face to the sky and let those wonderful drops trickle down my cheeks. I want to get soaked. I'll never complain about rain again."

I thought about how people didn't appreciate the small pleasures of life until they lost them. If I ever returned to a normal life, I'd enjoy every kind of weather, sunny or rainy, hot or cold. I'd remember the way it was in intensive care....

Chapter 10

I Figure It Out

"I have found it ! Eureka !"
Plutarch (46-120 A.D.)

In the morning when I awoke, I found I could lift my head and shoulders a couple of inches off the bed by contracting my upper back tapezius and deltoid muscles. However, the new movement didn't seem important because it really didn't change anything. I was still flat on my back and couldn't roll over or lift my arms. The fight to breathe dominated all other thoughts.

Today I wasn't assigned one of my special nurses. Rosa wasn't on duty and the others were either assigned to other patients or floating on other wards.

When my nurse began to change the sheets, she first lowered the head of my bed. That made it easier for her to move me up in the bed and get the sheet under me. Many other nurses also left my head lower than my feet as they moved me during sheet changing.

In that head down position, I still wondered whether gravity might cause the liquid food in my stomach to flow up my esophagus and then down into my trachea and lungs if the trach cuff wasn't fully inflated—since it often seeped air.

The thought that food effusion was contributing to my pneumonia led me to start signaling with my eyes for nurses to turn off the dripfeed before they lowered the head of my bed. Some got the message and turned off the dripline, but most didn't bother because they assumed the cuff was sealing well and there was no need.

When Dr. Sochat checked my lungs, he told me, "John, your right lung is still congested. The X-ray showed the same problem so I'd like to do another brochoscopy."

The last bronchoscopy went so smoothly that I quickly blinked my approval. I even enjoyed the last one when I got a chance to see inside my lungs.

The next morning, a different doctor came to do the bronchoscopy. I was not pleased because the first doctor had been skilled and I didn't know what to expect from this doctor. However, I was already committed.

The first procedure had been pleasurable with no discomfort, the second was totally wretched. One doctor was compassionate, the other indifferent. The ordeal made me realize how much doctors differed in their methods and their competency. If I needed any medical procedures in the future, I would be sure to request a doctor I was familiar with.

Chest X-rays in the following days showed the pneumonia persisted. The bronchoscopies had not accomplished anything. They had both been in vain. I wondered whether they were really necessary or whether they were done to give the doctors training in the procedure. Besides the discomfort involved, there had been the dangers of tissue damage, hemorrhaging, and lung collapse.

When a third bronchoscopy was advised, I refused. Dr. Sochat tried to persuade me, but I knew bronchoscopies for me were pointless until the source of my pneumonia was discovered. Meanwhile, the need for hourly suctioning continued.

As I tried to figure out the cause of my pneumonia, I remembered thinking that accumulated condensation in the ventilator tubing might somehow be directly entering my lungs through the trach tube. But how?

I recalled I sometimes became extremely dizzy when I was turned onto my right side. The ventilator was on my left so when turned to my right, the tubing was stretched to its limit and I could feel it pulling on my tracheostomy. In that stretched flat condition, any condensation that had pooled in the hanging loop was now free to flow directly into my trachea. That rush of water into my lungs could account for the dizziness—and maybe the pneumonia.

It began to make sense to me that my continuing pneumonia was either due to the effusion of my liquid food or from ventilator condensation—or both.

I wasn't absolutely sure I was right, and if my theory was wrong, I'd look foolish if I mentioned it. Even if I was right, I didn't think anyone would listen to me. I also didn't want to alienate the staff by calling attention to their oversights if it were true.

My thoughts bounced back and forth on whether to mention it to Dr. Sochat or not. I decided I would. I spelled out to him on the alphabet board as best I could that the dripfeed should be turned off before lowering the head of my bed and the ventilator tubes drained before turning me or moving me in a way that stretched the tubing taut.

It was a lot to spell out one letter at a time and I wasn't sure he understood the whole message, but the situation seemed to improve after I told him. Some nurses turned off the dripfeed before lowering my head and were careful about stretching the ventilator tubing when turning me on my right side.

The liquid food was nourishing me so I didn't have hunger pangs, but I had an overwhelming desire to eat real food. I wanted to smell, taste, and chew real food. My desire became an obsession, but wanting to eat was pointless because I hadn't been able to swallow since the paralysis began. With no air passing through my nose, I also had lost the ability to smell and taste.

Until now, I never realized the psychological importance of eating. It wasn't just a physical need. The sights, the smells, the tastes, and chewing were all part of the eating experience.

My craving to eat was triggered by food commercials on television. Using the prices in some supermarket commercials, I precisely calculated the total cost of preparing each meal to see how cheaply I could make them. It was good mental exercise and I also didn't know if I'd be broke when I got out of the hospital so I hoped I had enough money left to have one good meal. Just one good meal was all I wanted.

For hours at a time, I thought about cool watermelon juice trickling down my parched throat. I imagined myself slowly chewing a juicy steak, a baked potato smothered in butter, bacon and eggs, and turkey dinners with all the trimmings. I mentally savored each bite.

But, more than steak or fancy meals, I craved a chilidog smothered in onions and cheese. The juicy flavor of a hot dog, the spiciness of chili, the sharp taste of onions, and the soft, warm bun were obviously the greatest food created by man!

I worried that thoughts of eating might worsen my effusion problem. With no gag reflex and my trach cuff not sealing, I believed stimulating my salivary glands might cause the extra saliva to drain into my lungs.

Not having chewed for months, I also was concerned that poor blood circulation in my gums might lead to gingivitis, so I did a daily exercise to stimulate my gums. Since I could move my lower jaw, I firmly pressed my bottom teeth against my upper teeth to simulate chewing. I repeated the exercise for a few minutes, hoping the pressure would keep my gums firm and healthy.

Besides that brief physical exercise, I knew I also should do mental exercises. I needed to do more than watch television and count the holes in the ceiling tiles to keep my mind active. I worried that my mind would deteriorate if I just let it freewheel without any discipline. My mental faculties were intact and I wanted to keep them that way.

I wondered whether my mind would deteriorate without normal use. I had heard it said many times that the mind was like a muscle and you had to "use it or lose it." Neural connections might become dysfunctional from inactivity and cause networks to uncouple and disassociate, similar to aging. In addition, I wondered if my neural networks could become distorted by an overlay of mindless mental activity like excessive TV watching.

In any case, I was sure it was necessary to stay mentally active. The only question was how? Studying the Spanish chart Hugh had made was one way, but I needed more than that. I needed to devise personal mental exercises to keep my mind constructively busy during the day.

I devised memory exercises that were fun. I tried to recall the names of long-ago highschool classmates and former co-workers. I tried recalling as many state and country capitols and U.S. presidents as I could remember. The ones I couldn't recall kept my memory busy in the following days and weeks.

To maintain mental quickness, I pictured my fingers typing made-up sentences as fast as I could. Having played the piano for many years, I mentally fingered the chords to songs I had played in the past and "heard" the sounds in my mind's ear.

To exercise my reasoning powers, I compared how different philosophers would describe abstract concepts like truth and reality. I created math problems and did the calculations in my mind.

These mental exercises challenged my mind and served to temporarily divert attention away from my problems, but it was becoming difficult to maintain a positive outlook whenever I thought about my lack of significant physical improvement. I had been in the hospital for over two months and, except for a few minor, disconnected movements, I was basically the same as when I entered.

It was the belief that my recovery would turn a "sharp corner" that kept my hopes alive. The paralysis had happened quickly so I wanted to believe it would reverse itself as quickly as Dr. Hanson had told me it would. I reasoned, "My motor nerves lost their covering in two days, so once the reverse process starts, the covering will regenerate in two days." It made perfectly good sense to me. I wanted to turn that sharp corner as soon as possible so I could breathe, walk, and be the person I used to be.

I wouldn't admit to myself that my hope might be an illusion I created to make my life bearable. Had I simply suspended reality in the same way I suspended reality while watching a movie?

For the time being, I allowed the belief in a swift recovery replace logic. The reality of a lengthy, drawn out recovery was too much to face squarely, so I held on to my illusion. In my mind, my present slow progress was just a prelude to a swift turnaround.

My illusion was useful because it worked. It comforted me and allowed me to maintain a hopeful state of mind. It gave me an inspiring vision to focus on. I could say to myself, "It will happen soon John, hang in there."

I didn't stop to analyze that my unused muscles were shriveling up and atrophying. From my original weight of 190 pounds of firm muscle, I had deteriorated to 140 pounds of soft flesh. My former 32-inch waist was bloated like a big balloon and when the nurses turned me, I could hear the liquids sloshing around inside. The muscled biceps that formerly did heavy curls were now shapeless and weak. The legs that had squatted with hundreds of pounds were now thin and useless.

This was the body I somehow expected to get up and move when my motor nerves began functioning again. It wasn't logical, but it was my hope and I clung to it. I didn't even want to think about how my debilitated muscles might require months or possibly years of physical therapy.

My thoughts were interrupted by the arrival of Dr. Marshall and two of his staff. They went directly to the ventilator control panel and began talking in whispered tones so I wouldn't hear what they were saying. Nevertheless, I was able to hear enough to know there was a problem.

Someone had turned the ventilator up to 14 breaths a minute with 35% oxygen. They didn't know who, but it should not have been done. Dr. Marshall was upset by the tampering. He left the tidal volume at 700 ml, but turned the breaths back down to 12 at 23% oxygen.

Although I wished he would not adjust the ventilator controls, there was something about him that gave me confidence in him. I instinctively felt he knew what he was doing. That knowledge kept me reasonably calm whenever he turned down the settings.

This time, after he readjusted the settings, he came to my bedside and said, "John, I re-set the ventilator—as I'm sure you can feel. You always seem to know when I do. I realize it will be a little harder for you to breathe for a while, but it had to be done. Right now you probably can't appreciate that and you're angry with me, but it was necessary. When you're better and on your feet again, I give you permission to punch me in the nose for putting you through all this."

He understood…. He truly understood what I was going through. He was doing what he had to do and what was best for me, yet he apologized. I was deeply touched and would always remember his humanity.

Chapter 11

The Alarm Is Silent

"There was silence deep as death,
And the boldest held his breath."
Thomas Campbell (1777-1844)

I trusted Dr. Marshall, but why were so many others allowed to touch the ventilator's controls? I didn't believe all of them were authorized or skilled enough to adjust such a critical piece of equipment. When doctors, nurses, and respiratory therapists stood in front of the control panel, I didn't know if they were adjusting the controls or just checking to make sure they were set correctly. I wondered which one of them had recently improperly set the controls.

My overactive imagination suspected everyone was toying with the controls. It sometimes felt like they had decreased my oxygen supply even when they hadn't. In my heightened state of anxiety, I knew my imagination could play tricks on my mind, so I had to be careful not to hyperventilate and start a panic attack.

The respiratory therapists performed a number of duties. Besides doing the tricky job of changing the ventilator tubes, they applied a heavy vibrator to my chest to break up the congestion, tested my breathing, and cleaned the ventilator.

That afternoon, the respiratory therapist who came to clean the ventilator appeared to be someone without much experience. He fumbled as he removed the glass jar to wipe off condensation inside. The alarm didn't sound, so I knew he had turned it off while he worked. I nervously wondered, "Will he empty the water out of the tubes and collection jar? Will he remember to turn the alarm back on when he's done?"

He finished cleaning the machine and left. I hoped he hadn't forgotten to turn the alarm back on.

On this particular day, the ventilator hose's connection to my tracheostomy was a loose fit. Earlier in the day, it had popped off when the pressure built up inside. When it disconnected, there was a ten second delay before the alarm sounded. Rosa heard the alarm and rushed over to slip the hose back onto my trach tube. It was unsettling, but it didn't cause me to lose many breaths.

About an hour after the respiratory therapist had gone, the hose popped off again, disconnecting me from the ventilator. I counted the ten second delay and waited to hear the alarm. It was quiet. I thought maybe I had counted too fast. I waited. Still no alarm. He had forgotten to switch it back on!

The nurses were all busy and not looking my way. Two were tending other patients, one was sitting at the desk doing paperwork, and Rosa was in the supply room. None were aware of my dangerous situation and I had no way to attract their attention.

The disconnected tube was lying on my chest only an inch away from my tracheostomy. The disconnection was barely noticeable.

A minute passed. I could feel the lack of oxygen starting to take effect. Strangely, I was completely calm. It was as if I had known all along it would end like this, as if it was inevitable that I would suffocate to death. Two minutes passed. I was slowly losing consciousness. I was in the midst of nurses, but they didn't know I was in serious trouble. No help would be coming. I knew I had only a short time to live.

I always wondered what dying would be like. Now I knew. Dying was easy; there was nothing to fear. The irony was that I was dying with nurses all around me. The situation was so ridiculous, I couldn't help seeing the humor in it.

As I slowly slipped into unconsciousness, a relaxing aura swept over me. I became drowsy and felt pleasantly relaxed. Endorphins were being released in my brain to deal with the trauma of dying. They brought on a soothing feeling of tranquility. I felt no panic. I was resigned to die.

I was now almost unconscious. I looked around at the nurses so near and yet so far. They didn't know I was slipping away. My last thought was, "Well, so long...."

Darkness..........................Nothing...
....
....
....

Very faint sounds......... a faraway voice.............. a louder voice..............

"john... John... **JOHN**."

It was Rosa's voice. I opened my eyes and saw her beautiful face. As my mind slowly cleared, I could see a group of people crowded around my bed, anxiously staring down at me. It was the Code Blue team.

After a few minutes, the AMBU bag stabilized my breathing and I was reconnected to the ventilator. One of the emergency doctors checked my vital signs. He was satisfied I was stable. The emergency team left as quickly as they had come. I was back.

I didn't know what happened after I lost consciousness. I wasn't sure how I was found in time to prevent death or serious brain damage. Did the heart monitoring electrodes taped to my chest sound an alarm? Had Rosa found me unconscious when she routinely checked on me, applied the AMBU bag, and called the Code Blue team? Had they used the defibrillator or some other heroic measure to resuscitate me?

I had many unanswered questions, so I used the alphabet board to ask Rosa what had happened. She carefully dodged my question. The whole staff was extremely careful not to talk about the respiratory therapist's error. They obviously wanted to avoid an investigation and filling out reports. I doubted an incident report had been filed, and even if one had been filed, it would become part of the peer review process that neither myself nor anyone else had access to. Since no permanent harm had been done, they must have decided it was better to pretend nothing had happened.

Later that evening, the respiratory supervisor came into the ward and I overheard him quietly say to the headnurse, "I heard one of my people caused a problem this afternoon."

The headnurse whispered, "Yes, he was told about it." That was the last time anyone ever mentioned it.

As I thought about it, I wondered why I hadn't had either a near-death or an out-of-body experience. I simply had lost consciousness and then there was darkness.

People I had seen on television told of out-of-body experiences in which their minds rose up and looked down at their bodies below. Others described near-death experiences with vivid stories of seeing a brilliant white light, a long tunnel, and visions of dead relatives who spoke to them. The details of their stories were amazingly alike.

But, I had read about astronauts who had similar experiences while spinning around on a centrifuge. They lost consciousness and experienced a floating sensation, seeing a bright light at the end of a long tunnel, and unusual visions. Their experiences were remarkably similar to people who described their "near-death" experiences.

Physicians who analyzed the astronauts' experiences said the extreme G-force pressures prevented the normal flow of blood to their brains. The lack of oxygen caused cells to shut down with a brilliance like a dying supernova star. The massive cell firing created a bright light that was densest at the center, forming the illusion of a tunnel. The doctors labeled it "the dying experience" rather than "the near-death experience." They said the phenomena described by the astronauts were the normal progression of the body shutting down its functions, one by one.

The people who described their "near-death" experiences had probably gone through the same early stages of the "dying experience," but hadn't actually been near death. I didn't blame them for refusing to accept the physical explanation and clinging to the belief that it had been a spiritual experience.

I felt the same way. I wanted to believe in an afterlife too. It gave credence to the belief there was a part of me that would live on after death. It opened the door to that mysterious world I imagined was better than the one I was in. I also wanted to believe there was more to life than a short, troubled time spent on earth. I didn't want to accept death as the end of my existence either. I wanted to believe I had a spiritual self. The belief in the near-death experience offered "evidence" of a spiritual life after death and validated religion's promise.

But, I also knew that the mind was a wondrous organ that was capable of creating incredible visions and had an unlimited ability to believe in whatever it wanted to—or needed to—believe in. Nevertheless, we all had the right to our personal beliefs and no one could be proven wrong for their beliefs.

After carefully analyzing my two dying experiences, first in the isolation booth when I gave up, and the second when the ventilator hose disconnected, I began to understand more clearly what had occurred in each situation. My confusion gave way to a recognition of what had actually happened.

When I experienced a euphoric state in the isolation booth after letting go, I had been desperately ill, fighting for my life, and choking on my own fluids as I struggled for every breath. My brain was programmed by nature to deal with the trauma by releasing endorphins, a natural opiate, to ease the suffering. Endorphins produced a euphoric state of mind. In that dreamlike state, I felt a floating, drifting sensation as a way of separating my mind from my suffering body. No more, no less.

But, I asked myself why I hadn't experienced the same thing when the ventilator became disconnected and I had lost consciousness. There was no euphoria, no white light nor tunnel. I clearly remembered blacking out, then being wakened by Rosa and the Code Blue team. Why hadn't the lack of oxygen to my brain caused a dying experience? Why hadn't I experienced something?

I carefully thought about what had occurred and concluded I had been unconscious for only a couple of minutes and hadn't reached a condition of severe oxygen deprivation. I had merely blacked out in a faint. Cells had not yet begun to shut down. If the lack of oxygen had continued beyond that point, the dying experience with visions of a bright light and a tunnel would have begun. I hadn't reached that stage because I was resuscitated too quickly.

One thing I learned from my two experiences was that there was no suffering and no fear in the final moments of dying. The brain's endorphins created a tranquil state to deal with the trauma. Dying was like drifting off to a pleasant sleep. Nature designed it so.

Chapter 12

Why *Not* Me, God?

"God helps them that help themselves."
Benjamin Franklin

Charlene and Chris visited less often as the weeks passed. Sometimes it was a month between visits. However, my good friend Hugh came every week, often twice a week. He was my only real connection with the outside world.

I had a new visitor, the hospital priest. He had found that I was a Catholic from reading my file and came to introduce himself.

"John, I'm Father Hunkler. I just wanted to see how you were doing. Now that I'm familiar with your situation, I'll be visiting you until you're able to attend Sunday mass. In the meantime, I'll say a prayer for you every day. If there is anything that I can do for you, please let the nurses know and they'll get in touch with me."

He closed his eyes and said a silent prayer.

Father Hunkler kept his promise and often came to talk with me and offer solace. I appreciated his comforting visits, but I still didn't pray for God to cure me. I didn't think it was right to seek divine intervention whenever a misfortune occurred. I thought about what George Bernard Shaw had written, "Common people do not pray, they only beg." I continued praying without begging.

Neither did I ask, "Why me God?" Why *not* me? Was I special and exempt from disease? I had to play the cards I was dealt. There was no point in praying for a divine miracle or wishing it had happened to someone else instead of me. Whatever was happening to me was one of life's misfortunes and I had to deal with.

I also didn't believe my illness happened because I had somehow offended God. People who had serious diseases often believed they were being punished for having sinned and if they prayed to God, they'd be forgiven and their sicknesses would be miraculously cured. Guilt weighed heavily on their consciences and added to their depression if their prayers were not answered.

I didn't have that burden of guilt. I could accept my illness as a result of handling toxic chemicals—nothing more than that. It had nothing to do with punishment for having sinned. Eliminating guilt was one less problem I had to deal with and I felt better for it.

An hour after Father Hunkler left, Hugh arrived. I could see he was in a serious mood. He wanted to discuss my crumbling financial situation.

"John, your home is in danger of foreclosure, but I have a plan. I think we should move your furniture and belongings into storage. Then we can rent your house and use the money to pay some bills. At the same time, I can work with Charlene to sell your house in San Diego and that should keep you solvent for awhile. What do you think?"

His suggestion sounded like a workable plan so I blinked once.

"Okay then, that's what I'll do. After I get all your stuff into storage, I'll tell Charlene to advertise your house for rent and the other for sale."

It was difficult to understand why Hugh was doing all this for me. Packing and moving my things would be a huge job. I was immensely grateful to him for his help, but his offer of assistance was another reminder of how helpless and dependent I was on others.

The next morning, a new doctor came to introduce himself. It was time for Dr. Sochat to rotate to his next assignment and his replacement to take over. Dr. Sochat was another fine young medical intern and I'd miss him.

"Good morning, John. I'm Dr.Jeffries. I'll be taking Dr. Sochat's place. You probably don't remember me because we were all kind of busy that night, but I was with Dr. Sochat in the emergency room the night you came in. Let me check you to see how you're doing."

He gave me a brief but thorough check and said he'd see me later. My first impression of this young medical intern was positive. I marveled at the quality of these new, young doctors. The next generation of doctors was something to be proud of.

Things kept changing around me, but not within me. I was still basically paralyzed from head to toe and struggling to breathe on a ventilator.

My situation couldn't have been more miserable. It was as if some evil force had decided to torture me by taking away my ability to move, breathe, and speak—but left my sensory nerves intact so I could feel all the pain without being able to do anything about it. My emotions had built up to an intense level and wanted to be released. Tears of bitter frustration often welled up in my eyes, but I didn't dare tear up because that caused more fluid to accumulate in my nose and throat. I desperately wanted to cry to release the tension, but I had to hold it all in. I had no outlet for my feelings, no way to drain away even a little frustration.

During all the months of pure hell, I never once wondered why it happened to me and not someone else, but at one point I did think about whom I'd change places with if I could magically do it. Whom did I dislike enough to exchange my suffering for his health? I thought about it, but I couldn't think of one person in the world I hated so much that I'd wish this horror on him. It was too terrible to wish on anyone, no matter how much I disliked them. I never considered it again.

Sleep was my only escape. When I awoke, my eyes were often stuck shut with dried secretions, my nose ran, and my scalp and whole body itched. There was never a time when I was completely comfortable. If I had an itch, I automatically tried to move my hand to scratch it, but I couldn't. When I got tired of lying in one position, I unconsciously tried to roll over, but couldn't. My mind was a prisoner inside my frozen body. I tried to discipline my mind not to fight against the discomforts, but I didn't know how long I could keep control of my thoughts and hold on to my sanity. Sometimes it felt as if my mind was going to burst from the pressure.

A young woman in a white doctor's jacket was talking to Theresa and I heard the headnurse refer to her as a psychiatrist. I needed to talk to her.

Rosa was nearby and I caught her attention with my eyes. Using the alphabet board, I spelled out in pidgin English, "Want her" as I shifted my gaze to the psychiatrist.

She came over as soon as Rosa gave her the message. Smiling warmly, she greeted me, "Hello, the nurse said you wanted to see me. My name is Dr. Finch."

Rosa handed her the alphabet board. I spelled out, "Mind in trouble."

She asked, "What makes you think that?"

"Trapped."

"I'd feel trapped too if I was in your place. It's a difficult situation to be in. But, believe me, if you were in serious psychological trouble, you wouldn't be talking with me this way. You'd be acting much differently."

That's exactly what I wanted to hear. It made me feel a little better. Using the alphabet board, I spelled out as best I could, one letter at a time, the frustration of having an active mind trapped inside a paralyzed body.

Dr. Finch began probing into my negative feelings. However, the last thing I needed was an intense analysis that focused on the depressing aspects of my situation. I wasn't ready for that. Even though she was doing what psychiatrists are trained to do, at this time what I needed was encouragement and support. I needed her assurance that things weren't hopeless. I needed her to tell me I'd be okay—but she didn't. When she left, I felt worse.

Dr. Finch came back the following day and continued where she left off. She kept focusing on the negative side of my situation. After twenty minutes of probing, she said, "When your nerves heal, your muscles will be like limp spaghetti and you'll have to relearn how to do even the simplest things."

That did it. I couldn't take it anymore. The last thing I needed to hear was how helpless I was and what a terrible future lay ahead. She didn't understand I needed emotional support—not a searing analysis.

I spelled out, "Go."

My message startled her. She was obviously upset by it.

"Why John? Can't we talk some more?"

I closed my eyes, ending the conversation.

Before she left she said, "When you're better and able to speak, let me know what I did wrong."

She was just doing what she had been trained to do, but she somehow didn't realize the desperate situation I was in and what my needs were at that particular time.

Dr. Finch respected my wishes and I never saw her again. However, I later found out she kept in close touch with my doctors and nurses and worked with them without my knowing. This wonderful young psychiatrist hadn't deserted me. For many months, she secretly followed my situation and provided psychological advice to the staff. When they complained to her about my refusals of some treatments, she wrote in her report, "Being demanding and noncompliant are his only expressions of frustration, despair, loneliness, and pain. In fact, he has acted out minimally."

I wished I had had a chance to thank her after I learned of her participation, but it was only later that I became aware of all the subtle, unseen care she and so many other people gave that helped me enormously! If only I had known about all of their care and concern behind the scenes....

That afternoon, Dr. Marshall came in and turned my ventilator's sigh volume down to 1100 ml, but I didn't think of it as due to my improvement because it meant I was receiving less oxygen. This time Dr. Marshall gave me no speeches, he just quietly reset the machine and left. He figured I knew the score by now and I'd have to deal with it on my own. I could now, at times, trigger as many as 12 extra breaths a minute—but I didn't know it!

Despite the improvements I had made in breathing, I still felt short of oxygen because of the weaning process. My anxiety led me to spell out to Dr. Jeffries that I was having breathing problems. He immediately drew blood and sent it to the lab to check my blood gases. More blood drawings followed. All the results showed everything was normal. I never complained again because I knew it would put me through another series of painful blood drawings.

Various staff people drew my arterial blood gas samples: RNs, LVNs, lab personnel, and sometimes doctors. It was startling to see the different levels of competency. My arteries had sunk so deeply into my flaccid flesh, it was becoming more and more difficult to find an artery. Some nurses needed only one stick while others required many. Some weren't able to find the artery at all. Good nurses were not too proud to ask for help rather than subject me to numerous painful probes.

For three months I hadn't used most of my muscles and I worried some would atrophy and become permanently unusable. My reproductive system was no different. I was aware that my penile muscles could atrophy just like any other muscle.

I worried that my body was producing seminal fluids and was storing them without being able to release the pressure by ejaculating. I wondered how long it would be before the glands producing the reproductive fluids suffered internal damage or stopped functioning entirely. I wanted to preserve whatever functions I could. (Little did I know that Mother Nature placed my system in a suspended state that allowed the non-used organs to remain healthy and retain their functions).

Meanwhile, there were slight improvements in other areas. My latest movement was the ability to slightly shift my hips by contracting my abdomen and lower back. I could also slightly contract my biceps.

But once again, these small, isolated movements didn't excite me because they were overridden by the fact I still couldn't move a major muscle group that allowed me to do anything useful. I couldn't make any meaningful movements like turning my whole body, moving my arms or legs, or sitting up. I couldn't talk, swallow, or breathe. Basically, I remained paralyzed with only small, isolated movements in a few unconnected areas. I remained totally dependent on the nurses.

I further worried my progress might totally stop at some point and leave me bedridden for the rest of my life. What was my future? Would I ever recover or would I end up a human vegetable, a paralyzed bed patient for the rest of my life?

Charlene visited that evening. She had put one of my houses up for sale and received an offer. She held the paper so I could read it. The offer was ridiculously low. The potential buyer was probably aware that I was in the hospital and desperate to sell. I needed to sell the house so I could make payments on the other two I owned, but I wasn't willing to sell at a give-away price. I blinked twice for "No." Charlene agreed with me and said she would give them my rejection.

It was difficult to concentrate on business when my real focus was on my physical problems. The outside world seemed a million miles away.

It was time for Dr. Jeffries to rotate to a new assignment. A new doctor would be taking over my care. She came the next day. Dr. Unger was a small, thin young woman, who didn't say much but seemed capable. She made the usual checks of my vital signs and left.

After she left, I received good news. The headnurse Theresa told me she had decided to keep me in ICU a while longer. Though I was still on a ventilator, I had been in ICU for almost four months and was suitable for transfer to a rehabilitation ward. I guessed the staff had formed a closeness with me and wanted to keep me as long as they could.

As it turned out, Theresa's decision probably saved my life. A regular ward would not have the one-to-one nursing I had in intensive care. Nurses would be in a distant station and not immediately available. Ventilator problems, critical suctionings, and other major problems would have had disastrous consequences on a regular ward. I would not have survived.

Chapter 13

Power Misused Is Power Abused

"A wise man never refuses anything of necessity."
Publius Syrus (42 B.C.)

It was July. Four months had passed since my paralysis began. Dr. Marshall reset the ventilator to 800 ml tidal volume at 10 breaths a minute with a 1100 ml sigh volume. He reduced the number of breaths because I could trigger up to 12 extra breaths per minute on my own—all of which was still unknown to me. More importantly, he set the oxygen level at 21% which was the normal room level. If I knew the significance of that, I might have been inspired, but no matter what the ventilator settings were, it was always a challenge to breathe—which was the plan of course, only I didn't know it. In my mind, it was the same old struggle.

My power to say "No" by rolling my head from side to side was proving to have its faults as well as its advantages. Not allowing the nurses to turn me at times had changed the red rash on my buttock to a stage one erythema that had the potential for becoming a decubitus. I also wrongly stopped the nurses from sitting me up in the cardiac chair. Though I hated the discomfort of the chair, in the long run it was good for me to get out of bed and sit erect, even for a short while. It took a lot of effort for the staff to get me into the chair and their willingness to do it showed good nursing.

Shaking my head or any other gesture I made was of no value if the staff didn't try to understand what it meant. My special nurses could almost read my mind, but others had trouble understanding.

One of the inexperienced student physical therapists didn't like it when I shook my head "No." I was trying to tell her to be careful when she moved me so she wouldn't stretch the ventilator tube taut and dump condensation directly down my trachea. She had no idea what I was trying to tell her. She scolded me for being a "bad patient" and turned me way over on my right side, unknowingly dumping ventilator water down my trachea and causing the dizzying sensation. She had no idea what she had done.

Though my headshaking power was small, I tried not to abuse it. Power was only good when used wisely. I refused a procedure only after I considered the consequences—sometimes I erred.

When I refused some treatments, a nurse wrote in her reports, "Mr. Sueta seems not to want to get well,. He is uncooperative in whatever manner he is capable."

I didn't understand how anyone could possibly believe I was not trying to breathe better and increase my movements? If I could trigger the ventilator to deliver more air by simply trying harder, why would I ask for higher oxygen settings and subject myself to painful blood drawings to justify it? The reality was that the ventilator was set at 10 breaths per minute and I could trigger more only when my strength was high and conditions were right, but I couldn't sustain the effort for long periods of time.

Any criticism exemplified the different "realities" that often existed between staff and patients. Anyone who thought I was not trying to improve was accusing me of the "patient's dilemma," which occurred when a patient wanted to remain at a level that had become comfortable rather than struggle to reach the next level of recovery. It didn't apply to me because I was definitely not at a comfortable level. Trapped in a paralyzed body, struggling for every breath, and battling constant pneumonia was not a "comfort zone" that I chose to remain in. I was fighting with every ounce of strength I had to get better and any staff member who didn't believe that had unrealistic expectations that were counter-productive.

My present intern, doctor Unger, also vented her frustration of my slow progress because it didn't meet her expectations, the "big E." She felt her best efforts weren't being met with my best efforts, that my seeming noncooperation was holding back my progress. Her limited experience hadn't yet taught her how to work with the normal flow of a patient's recovery with its ups and downs. She hadn't yet learned to accept the periods when a patient's progress temporarily leveled off and hit a plateau. My chart obviously showed my improvement was slow but steady. (Months later, I met Dr. Unger on another ward and she told me,"You were my favorite patient." In spite of our differences, she understood me later and had developed a respect for my attempts to participate in my own care).

But, my own expectations were unrealistic too. I still wanted to believe my paralysis would "turn a sharp corner" and quickly reverse. I still held onto that false expectation.

The only good news I had during August was I could slightly flex the quadriceps muscles on the front of my thighs. It didn't occur to me that one day these minor, isolated movements might connect to form larger, important movements. I wished someone had brought it to my attention! My mind was too involved in my more immediate problems.

Charlene visited in the afternoon with a buyer's counter-offer to buy my beach house. It wasn't a fair offer, but I needed cash immediately to pay bills that were long overdue. I blinked once in acceptance of the offer and Charlene left immediately to get the sale in motion. The sale would temporarily ease my financial woes, but wouldn't last if I stayed too long in the hospital.

I felt a heavy sadness in losing this wonderful property near the ocean that I had planned to build condos on one day. I had even designed them and made full architectural drawings. It was another part of my former life that was gone forever.

Charlene and Chris visited me less often as time passed. Now they came only once a month. It really didn't matter to me because no matter how many visitors I had, they represented a very small part of my life as a patient. Ninety-nine percent of my time was spent with the nurses. They were my world. They were there when everyone else had gone home.

My ventilator remained my major source of anxiety. Too many people had access to the control panel and I was certain some tampering by inexperienced people caused wrongful settings—which in fact had happened. When Dr. Marshall came by, I used the alphabet board to ask him if he would put tape over the alarm button and other controls to stop unauthorized people from tampering. He understood my anxiety and put tape marked "Do Not Change" over critical knobs.

I relaxed and felt much better. People still had access to the controls, but at least the safety alarm was on and the main settings were protected.

My relief was short lived. The first respiratory therapist who came by, not knowing who had placed the tape, removed it and I was back to square one.

It was time again for a new doctor. Until now, I had been lucky. Today my good luck changed. My new doctor was a young woman with an attitude problem. From the outset, she was extremely aggressive and unfriendly.

Dr. Bodin introduced herself. She saw the alphabet board and picked it up to talk. I needed suctioning, so I spelled out, "suction."

She glared at me and sarcastically said, "I'm not a nurse."

I knew right away I was going to have a problem with her.

I figured she was either overcompensating for her lack of confidence by showing she was in charge or else she thought she had to prove she was as tough-minded as her male counterparts. Whatever the cause, we were off to a bad start.

She decided to take a blood sample. I shook my head "No" because it had been done only the day before.

She proceeded to intimidate me with dire warnings of diseases that were going around the hospital and a blood sample was absolutely necessary. After her repeated bullying, I gave in. Her technique was as aggressive as her attitude. Instead of using my arm, she drew blood from my femoral artery, which was extremely more painful than taking it from my arm.

She left with the sample. I wasn't looking forward to our next meeting.

My type of paralysis was quite rare, so many doctors came by to observe me. Some were neurologists, but most were medical students coming to observe my unusual disease.

One neurology resident stopped by a few times. During a visit, he felt compelled to tell me, "With Guillain Barré, you'll recover some function, but you'll always have some residual paralysis." He then proceeded to give me his pessimistic predictions about my future recovery with its limitations. He wasn't being malicious, he thought he was being forthright and giving me useful information.

After he left, I was despondent. The young doctor's negative comments bothered me for days. His words painted a gloomy picture of my future and I couldn't stop thinking about what he had said. As with Dr. Finch, the psychiatrist, I needed encouraging words more than a demoralizing prognosis.

I knew that many doctors were inclined to tell patients the worst. Common statements were, "You'll never walk again," or "You won't be the same person you were." Why did doctors make such gloomy predictions before they fully considered the effects they would have on patients?

Most were said at a time when there was no reason to say anything at all. They were said before doctors really understood the situation and before patients were ready to hear such crushing predictions. Were these doctors playing it safe in case patients didn't improve as expected? Were they describing the worst case scenario so they wouldn't be criticized for an optimistic prediction that didn't work out? (The American Medical Association states, "If no questions are asked, knowledge should not be forced upon the patient.")

Whether or not to dispense a negative prognosis was one of the many "doctors' dilemmas." I understood there were times when it was obvious a patient would not improve and it was wrong to give false hope. But, in my case, there was no clear understanding of how much I would recover and therefore, no medical opinion was called for.

Furthermore, there was no harm in allowing me to remain optimistic, no matter what the outcome might be. Hope was all I had and no one had the right to take it away from me. Hope gave me a reason to keep on keeping on. The bleak picture painted by the young doctor served no purpose whatsoever and could have been left unsaid. Why force it on me? Making no prediction would have been the kindest thing to do because, "Hope once crushed, is less quick to spring again."

The neurology resident who dispirited me should have first learned more about my condition before being so brutally candid. He should have acquired that knowledge by carefully observing me over a longer period of time, not from a few brief visits. He could have emphasized the positive aspects rather

97

than the negative. He could have explained the seriousness of my condition while assuring me that everything possible was being done, phrasing it in a way that left the door open for hope.

It had been a bad day and it got worse. That afternoon the patient in the next bed went into cardiac arrest. Theresa called the Code Blue team. Within minutes, a team of doctors, nurses, and RTs came running into the ward. In a frenzy of activity, CPR was started, injections given, and a messy bedside operation was performed. The noise and wild disorder went on for almost an hour.

With the frenzied excitement happening so near, I had an anxiety attack. The emergency in the next bed had caused me to fight the ventilator. I didn't know what was happening to me except that I couldn't breathe. My panicked attempts to breathe interfered with the ventilator's cadence and caused the alarm to begin beeping wildly, but no one heard it because of all the noise and confusion in the next bed.

Somehow in the chaos, Theresa looked over at me and saw I was in trouble too. She grabbed the AMBU bag, disconnected me from the ventilator, and pumped oxygen into me until I was ready to be reconnected to the ventilator.

In the next bed, the emergency team left when the patient couldn't be saved. It had been an extremely stressful incident.

The next day, I heard about a coming change that further dismayed me. I overheard nurses talking about two ICU nurses who were transfering to other wards. As I listened more carefully, I heard the names Gary and Rosa. Both of them were leaving me! The news came as a complete shock because I hadn't expected it and I had grown to depend on them so much. I wouldn't have their special care anymore.

Later that afternoon, Gary came to my bedside to say goodbye.

"Well, John, I'm sure you've heard that I'll be leaving ICU. I was offered a promotion to headnurse on an intermediate care ward and I've decided to accept it. I'll still be around and I promise to stop in and see you from time to time. You're coming along well so I want you to hang in there and keep on fighting the good fight."

He took my limp hand in his and I said goodbye with my eyes. And then he was gone.

A short while later, Rosa came to tell me about her new assignment. "John, did you hear that I'm transferring to an intermediate care ward on the next floor?"

I blinked once.

"I need to get a break from the crazy pace here in ICU. Most nurses don't stay too long in intensive care because it's too physically and mentally demanding. There are some nurses who prefer working in ICU and the ER because they like the excitement and the adrenalin rush, but it's hard for a lot of nurses to be emotionally challenged all the time and still keep their mental balance."

After she said that, I understood why many of the nurses in ICU were young. It wasn't a place most nurses stayed for a long time.

She chatted with me for a while, then said before she left, "John, I promise to stay in touch and visit you whenever I can. I'll be seeing you soon, I promise."

Rosa was a very wise young woman. I understood what she meant about nurses needing to protect their emotional well-being. I didn't blame her for leaving intensive care, though I'd miss both her and Gary more than they realized. I said goodbye to Rosa with tear-filled eyes.

Rosa made me think about the incredible stresses faced by nurses. Nursing was a job filled with wonderful highs and terrible lows.

One advantage nurses had over me was they could leave the hospital and go home, relax, and recharge their batteries before returning to face another stressful day. They could shop at the mall, eat out, and take in a movie. However, I couldn't escape my stressful situation. I had to live in that small bed twenty-four hours a day with no relief, no way to get away from the relentless stress even for a minute.

For days, my ears had been slowly clogging up with coagulated wax. Now they were totally closed. All I could hear was the throbbing of my pulse on my eardrums. My eyes watered constantly and the saltiness stung and made them water even more. The secretions caked up and completely blocked my vision. Now I couldn't see nor hear. My inability to breathe had eliminated my senses of smell and taste. I was left with no sights, no sounds, no smells or tastes. These senses were gone. The only sense I had left was touch.

The silent darkness felt as if I was entombed in a coffin. I was familiar with sensory deprivation experiments where people who had all their senses blocked, hungered for sensory stimulation so badly their minds hallucinated to create false sights and sounds. The silence and darkness was forcing me into the same internal world of stimulus hunger and I feared I'd begin hallucinating.

Sometime later, I didn't know how long, I felt someone gently shaking me. I tried to open my eyes but couldn't see through the caked-on material covering them. It was Dr. Bodin. She saw my eyes were clogged, so she carefully wiped them with wet tissues until I could see.

She sensed something else was wrong and picked up the alphabet board. I spelled out, "No hear." She responded immediately by getting an irrigation kit from the storeroom and proceeded to clear my ear canals with a syringe filled with a cleansing solution.

Once the months of accumulated wax was flushed from my ears, I could hear again. Seeing and hearing allowed me back into the real world of ICU. It was a world of misery, but it was all I had.

Chapter 14

Seeking A Partnership

"All your strength is in your union,
All your danger is in discord."
Henry Wadsworth Longfellow

When September rolled around, it was time for a new doctor to be assigned. I wasn't sorry to see Dr. Bodin leave. (However, as happened so often, I only saw part of the picture and my sense of reality was flawed. Things are seldom what they seem---even when you're absolutely sure you are right. I learned later how much support she had actually given me. Many months later when I read her reports, I developed a whole new feeling about her. I learned she had been trying to understand my refusals of treatments and my nonsubmissive attitude. It had been difficult for her to accept my behavior, so she countered with forceful doctoring—the only way she believed she could accomplish the things necessary to do her job. If I didn't submit to frequent blood tests and X-rays, she felt she couldn't properly monitor my condition. Initially, she had been uncompromising, but later she mellowed and wrote in my records, "Patient is an intelligent man, his refusals are his only means of controlling his life's events ... he will allow lab work when you give him impressive reasons for needing results...please try to minimize routine lab work." It took a little time, but she later understood. I felt she would become a good doctor after all. Unfortunately, I never had a chance to tell her so).

My refusals of some procedures were actually positive signs of my motivation to be involved in my care. I wasn't being difficult or manipulative. In the past, I had allowed the staff to use experimental antibiotics, perform two spinal taps, a thoracentesis, two bronchoscopies, many X-rays, and a large number of blood drawings. I mainly limited only the frequency of some procedures.

I was trying to have some control over my own body and do what I felt was best for me. For a long time I had no way of objecting to anything and I received aggressive care that I felt was sometimes unnecessary. Being a patient didn't mean I was a mindless lump of flesh that had to agree with everything the staff wanted to do. There were some procedures I felt were unnecessary and not in my best interests. If I had let the doctors have total control, I would probably have been X-rayed and had blood drawn every day. That would have been for their benefit, not mine. Too many X-rays were known to be dangerous and I had already had too much X-ray exposure, so I felt I had to limit them to a reasonable frequency. Blood drawings became extremely painful and often impossible to obtain. My black and blue arms looked like a drug addict's track marks, so I limited blood drawings to a frequency that still gave the staff enough information to set the ventilator and make decisions.

When the doctors and I disagreed about managing my care, who was right and who was wrong? Were the doctors always right and I was obligated to go along with whatever they wanted to do? On the other hand, should I have total control of what care I received? Did a "good" patient never question treatments? Refusing some treatments didn't automatically make me a "bad" patient. However, the mindset of some staff was they always knew what was best for me. They focused on my refusals and not the reasons behind them.

It presented the dilemma of whether to risk offending the staff by asserting my opinions on treatment or else to let them treat me in whatever way they chose. I decided to stay involved but never offend my caretakers. I owed the nurses and doctors my respect for their efforts to help me.

Many times, I had overheard staff members describe me as "alert and oriented." Since I was mentally alert, I felt I should be a partner in helping guide my care and the staff should have welcomed my input. We both had something to contribute.

Doctors only knew what was evident from tests. I knew what couldn't be seen by tests. I knew when I felt nauseous and needed medication, when I felt oxygen deprived and needed suctioning, when I needed a sedative, and many other internal things tests didn't show. Combining my input with their medical knowledge was the best course of action.

The one thing I sometimes abused was my objection to be turned so often. There were many reasons for not wanting to be turned. Lying on my side was more uncomfortable, but the nurses kept me on my side so much that I seldom had the relief of lying flat. More importantly, I couldn't breathe as well on my side because my chest expansion was restricted.

Another reason I didn't want to be turned so often was some nurses lowered my head when turning me and I still believed I might effuse food into my lungs if the dripfeed wasn't turned off and my trachea cuff wasn't sealing.

I was in a "catch 22" situation. If I didn't allow them to turn me frequently, I dared getting a decubitus. If I let them turn me, I couldn't breathe as well and there might be effusion from either the dripfeed or ventilator condensation.

Sometimes I won my point when I objected to a procedure, sometimes I lost. (I didn't know it at the time, but the Patient's Bill of Rights gave me "… the right to refuse treatment" and the AMA recognized, "a patient should be a partner in his own treatment and encouraged to exercise his right to complain").

At times, I was engaged in a psychological tug of war. Some staff were trying to pull me toward submissiveness while I was trying to pull them toward accepting me as a partner in my own care, respecting my decisions to limit some procedures. It became an intense contest of wills at times and it wasn't a fair fight. I was a lone, paralyzed patient, lying down, on a ventilator, and no match for a staff who had the ultimate power to control almost everything.

I couldn't speak to fully explain myself, so many of the staff didn't understand the deeper reasons for my refusals. Some of the staff believed I was refusing as a way to vent my emotions. One doctor reported, "Patient must be experiencing extreme difficulty with issues of control and may attempt to exert influence in the only way he sees as possible through apparent lack of cooperation with his treatment."

That was true sometimes. There were times when my fears and frustrations overwhelmed me and I had to release tension by acting out. I was only human, in an incredibly difficult situation, and sometimes I behaved like an obstinate jerk. But, those outbreaks didn't happen often. Some staff, like Dr. Bodin, understood my rationale only after dealing with me for a while.

Dr. Jeffries wrote in his report,"If you talk to the patient and explain what you want to do, you'll find you won't have too much difficulty." Some staff members admired my self-control under such extreme duress and my efforts to be a partner in my own care.

I remembered reading about Norman Cousins[1], the noted author and UCLA School of Medicine faculty member, who lived through two severe illnesses of spinal arthritis and a massive heart attack. As a patient he developed a working relationship with his doctors and became a partner in his care. He refused to take an angiogram, refused a coronary bypass operation, convinced his doctor to let him operate the treadmill himself, and engaged in strenuous exercise against his doctor's advice. He was not a patient that accepted all treatments and advice. He marched to a different drummer.

However, his doctors didn't regard his medical intrusions as meddling. They respected his self-responsibility. They worked together with him in a partnership. The symbiotic relationship gave Cousins a feeling of self-determination and the doctors learned the value of receiving input from a patient. The excellent results led many doctors to change their methods. Mr. Cousins lived another ten productive years of writing and teaching.

I had been unconsciously doing some of the things he had done as a patient. Our situations were not identical, but our efforts to control some of the treatments and work with the staff in a partnership were similar.

However, I had no say-so in my ventilator settings. Dr. Marshall had complete control. Though I didn't fully appreciate it at the time, it was definitely good he did because I might have demanded more oxygen and retarded the development of my inspiratory muscles. It was through my struggles to

---

[1] The Healing Heart, Norman Cousins, W.W. Norton & Co.,1983

inhale more air that forced my chest muscles to work harder and grow stronger.

I had no way to tell Dr. Marshall how much I believed in him. I believed in him so much that, as frightened as I was, I would have allowed him to turn the damn ventilator off if he said it was okay! That's how much trust a good doctor like him inspired.

Dr. Marshall reset my ventilator to 700 milliliters at 7 breaths a minute. The setting kept me working hard. As I labored to breathe, I unknowingly triggered as many as 16 extra breaths a minute, depending on my energy level.

My efforts to prevent the staff from causing excessive effusion seemed to be working and my pneumonia gradually improved until I didn't need suctioning quite so often. Since my pneumonia had abated, the antibiotic dripneedle in my foot was removed. Things were looking a little better, but my condition was still deplorable. The red rash on my buttock finally broke down and developed into a stage three decubitus. The soft, wet flesh was now an open sore that could easily grow into a large, infected ulcer. Now I could not be left on my back at all. It was all my fault.

Blood samples were getting difficult to take by everyone. I heard the doctors discussing a machine that could measure the amount of chemicals in my blood by shining a light through my earlobe.

I thought, "If only I had that machine, it would save me all these painful blood drawings."

A couple of days passed when I saw a lab doctor and two assistants wheel in a computer console. He explained the basics of the machine to them while he placed a small unit over my left ear and clamped it on my earlobe. He covered the earpiece with a black cloth to shut out external light. The team watched the digital readout on the console as they passed an infrared light source through my earlobe.

I waited, full of hope that blood tests would be minimized.

They had a reading! "John, the machine is working well. Your arterial oxygen saturation level is good. We'll leave the unit by your bed and use it from now on."

He looked into my eyes, silently telling me how glad he was that I wouldn't have to endure so many painful blood drawings.

My spirits were further raised when Hugh visited. He told me, "I talked with the manager of my engineering department about you and he said you can have some design work to do at home when you leave the hospital. You'll be back doing what you love to do."

That was music to my ears. It didn't really matter whether that would ever happen because just thinking of a return to my former life filled me with hope. It gave me a vision of a life beyond the troubled world I now lived in. It made me believe I might have a future. Hugh was a great friend who never stopped giving.

Giving also came from the Salvation Army. The wonderful volunteers in their dark blue uniforms came to the ward from time to time and distributed packages containing toiletries and other much needed items. They didn't expect anything in return. It was just part of their great work that went unnoticed.

Later that evening, Charlene came with a real estate agent representing a group of business people who had made the offer to buy my beach house. It figured. They were probably going to tear down the house and build condominiums on the land, just as I had planned to do. The nurses sat me up so I could read the forms and sign them. They put a pen between my teeth and I moved my head to make a crude mark which substituted for my signature.

I used the alphabet board to tell Charlene to use the money left over after expenses to pay all the overdue bills. My outside problems were temporarily taken care of, but I had no idea how long I could keep my bills paid if my hospitalization lasted the nine months or more the doctors predicted. Incredibly, the thought of losing everything didn't bother me that much. All I wanted was to get well and everything else seemed unimportant. It took a serious illness to show me what really mattered.

Days passed and things went along as usual until late August when a major change in my condition occurred. Norby, the male nursing aide, cranked up the head of my bed, propped pillows to hold me in place, and let me sit in an upright position. It felt good to be sitting up and breathing was easier with my lungs in a normal position.

The ventilator was now set at a low 700 milliliters with 6 breaths a minute at 21% oxygen. I was assisting and could trigger around 12 extra breaths a minute. Unknown to me, this was a perfect situation for breathing on my own without the ventilator. The parameters were all at the right levels, minimum tidal volume of 500 ml, breaths between 12 and 29, and oxygen percentage at normal room level.

Norby disconnected me from the ventilator while he suctioned my airways. He noticed I was breathing well without using the AMBU bag. After he finished suctioning me, he paused and didn't reconnect me to the ventilator like he usually did. Instead, he just stood by and watched me closely.

I wasn't sure what he was doing, but I felt okay. Norby waited calmly. I waited less calmly.

He was composed and said, "Let's stay this way for a minute."

I nodded my head. With good old Norby standing by, I felt confident I was in no immediate danger. I completely trusted him.

A minute passed.. two…three…four…five minutes passed.

Finally, I signaled with my eyes that I wanted to be reconnected. I was getting worried. This was a giant step and I wasn't sure if everything was okay. That ventilator had been my lifeline for five long months and my mind was still connected to it even though my body wasn't.

Still calm, Norby said, "Let's try another few minutes." He could tell by my skin color and breathing rate that I was getting enough oxygen. This was all being done by a "mere" nursing aide!

I was breathing through the trach tube so I still couldn't speak. I blinked once. I wanted to get off that damn machine—no matter what some of the staff believed! They said in their reports I was "ventilator dependent" and "not trying." How wrong they were. I wanted to breathe on my own more than they could ever know. I was controlling the situation now and taking responsibility for my own welfare. It was up to me whether I went back on the machine. I didn't want to go back and Norby knew it.

Ten minutes passed. I felt fine. Norby checked my blood pressure and pulse rate to make sure I wasn't having any problems.

A long half-hour went by. My breathing was shallow but adequate. A nursing aide had taken it upon himself to get me off the ventilator. I was breathing on my own!

Norby informed the staff of what was happening. No one interfered. Everyone just watched and waited. My skin color was observed for any sign of cyanosis and my vital signs were carefully monitored.

I was excited, but only time would tell if I had the endurance to continue breathing sufficiently on my own. I was determined to try. I noticed I could move my lip muscles enough to form a small smile for Norby.

An hour later, the afternoon shift came on duty. Norby had to leave and the new shift took over. I continued breathing on my own. I watched television but stayed fully vigilant of how well I was breathing, monitoring every breath.

Hours passed. The night shift came on duty. I was afraid to fall asleep. Whenever I did drop off, I awoke with a jolt and immediately checked my breathing.

The night doctor wasn't sure I should be off the ventilator and wanted to put me back on it, but I shook my head "No." I wanted to see if I could keep breathing on my own—and I did. All through the night and into the next morning, I breathed unassisted.

I was free! Unless something unforeseen happened, I was done with the ventilator for good. Maybe now, the staff people who didn't believe I had been trying hard, understood how wrong they were.

Since no one had explained to me how the weaning process was done, I didn't know if everything was going the way it was supposed to or not.

Dr. Marshall heard the news and stopped by to explain, "I'm really proud of you John. We had to keep the ventilator set at a minimal output that forced you to breathe harder and develop your chest muscles. If the ventilator had been set at a nice, comfortable level, you would have let the machine do everything and stayed dependent on it forever. It must have been hellish, but I'm sure you're glad we did what we had to do."

I blinked once and expressed my gratitude with my eyes.

I learned later that weaning a patient off a ventilator was normally a carefully controlled procedure. The standard method of weaning was lengthy and technical. It required medications, frequent blood gas analyses, checking vital signs every fifteen minutes, detailed data recording, and patient education. For nurses, it required exhaustive patience and effort. I was able to bypass all that, thanks to an excellent Dr. Marshall and an equally excellent nursing aide, Pat Norby.

Although I was off the ventilator, I still needed frequent suctioning through my tracheostomy and my major paralysis remained. More and more, I began to realize there might not be a sharp corner of recovery when my paralysis would quickly reverse itself. However, a part of me still needed to believe in a miraculous turnaround. The reality of a long recovery process was too difficult to accept.

I knew everyone had days of hope and days of despair. I had struggled with conflicting emotions before my illness too. I remembered past times when the difficulties of living had brought me to the point of sinking into the dark waters of depression. But, somehow I had always managed to come bobbing back up to the surface, swimming with renewed strength.

Chapter 15

Cutting the Umbilical Cord

"This was the most unkindest cut of all."
Julius Caesar, William Shakespeare

Now that I was off the ventilator, the doctor in charge of ICU decided they needed the bed I occupied for incoming patients. Theresa explained the situation to me, "John, tomorrow you'll be moving to a rehabilitation ward. I really hate to see you leave, but it's time for you to be on a rehab ward where they can give you special treatment. I've been told you'll be in a room with a window and have other patients for company. You'll receive good care there."

It was a sincere farewell. I was sure some of the staff would miss me as much as I would miss them, but the wheels of the hospital had to keep turning. Things change.

I would *not* miss the constant life-and-death struggle of patients around me, the radiation exposure from nearby patients being X-rayed, or a couple of the staff that didn't believe in me.

Some of the staff had grown tired of taking care of me. In the beginning, their interest in me had been high. I was a new challenge and most nurses had been attentive and gave me their best care. But, after six long months, some lost their original enthusiasm because of my extremely slow progress, my sometimes uncooperative attitude, and the large amount of care I required. My minor improvements didn't meet their expectations. I didn't offer enough positive reinforcement to justify their efforts. Those who weren't able to intrinsically reward themselves for my small improvements, justifiably lost their motivation.

Even two of my special nurses tapered down to giving only routine care. I understood. It was only normal that they couldn't maintain such a high level of motivation as the months dragged on. I noticed it in their decreased attention to the little things. Everyone has their limits. It demonstrated how nurses could burn out on a single patient even though they remained motivated with other patients. However, some of their enthusiasm did return after they had a chance to back off for a while and recharge their emotional batteries.

My enthusiasm also burned out from time to time. Many times I became discouraged with my minimal progress. When I got depressed, a few nurses didn't understand. I guessed they expected me to have a positive attitude at all times. Nurses would probably describe an "ideal" patient as one who was always cooperative and cheerful.

I found that being cheerful at all times was not only impossible, but it wasn't even desirable. I needed an outlet for my pent-up frustrations. Venting my anger was as necessary as any medical treatment. A few nurses didn't realize my anger was a natural emotion occurring in response to my frustration. Anger and frustration go together like ham and eggs. Instead of taking offense at my anger, nurses should have accepted the fact my anger showed I hadn't given up, that inside I still had the spirit to fight against my awful situation.

In normal life, when I got frustrated and angry, I could harmlessly vent my feelings by exercising or doing something physical that burned off the negative energy. Now I couldn't do anything except lie there and accumulate negative energy without having a way to release it.

My special nurses understood. Their written reports said, "…supported patient's emotions…allowed patient to vent… complimented patient's spirit." Many of my doctors were likewise understanding in their positive notes, describing my attitude as "justifiable." When I read their notes later, I was truly amazed that doctors and nurses who were young, in good health, and had never been in a helpless situation, could have such compassion for my psychological needs. I loved them for their understanding.

I didn't want to leave intensive care. I was familiar with the staff and the daily routine. There was comfort in knowing what to expect. Now I was going to an unfamiliar place I knew nothing about. The change was frightening because so much was unknown. I had no idea what the new ward would be like. I imagined it would be less frantic than the intensive care ward, but on the other hand, I wouldn't have one-to-one nursing care. There would be only a few nurses to take care of twenty or thirty patients. Would my suctioning be monitored as closely? Would I receive as much important nursing care? How would I adjust to the new surroundings and staff? Tomorrow I'd find out. It was time to leave the womb.

At nine o'clock the next morning, Theresa told me it was time to transfer. She and an aide put my hospital file, my possessions, and my potted plant in a box on the bed with me. As they wheeled me out, I turned my head and nodded "Goodbye" to the nurses. Norby, and Anne smiled and waved back. My home for the past six months would soon be only a memory.

We went through the swinging doors, down a series of hallways, and arrived at Ward 4-South. The headnurse who met us exchanged greetings with the ICU nurses.

I had been promised a room with a window and other patients to keep me company. I wasn't prepared for what came next. They wheeled me into a small, single-bed room, with no windows. It was dark and depressing. Theresa in ICU had been mistakenly informed about the room I would be in. Whether I liked it or not, I was here.

The headnurse was friendly and smiling as she welcomed me. The first thing she did was unpack the box and remove my file and personal possessions. They transferred me onto my new bed and set up my dripfeed. Once I was settled, Theresa smiled and said goodbye as she wheeled away my old bed. The headnurse straightened out my covers and shut the door behind her as she left.

Alone.... I was completely alone with no one within eyesight for the first time since I entered the hospital. In ICU's isolation booth, I had nurses nearby and I could see them through the booth's window.

I also didn't have heart monitors taped to my chest and there wasn't a call-button to push for help. There was nothing. The door was closed. I had no way to call for help. I could choke on my fluids and no one would even know.

"My god. There's no one here." I was struck with a terrible dread. I had never felt so alone and helpless in my life! How was I going to call for help if I needed suctioning? Would I choke on my own fluids if help didn't come quickly? Would I be turned every two hours? What about all the other things the nurses in ICU did for me?

I lay there in the silence, terrified, but still able to assess my situation. My pneumonia was gone, but my breathing was borderline and my immobility meant I still needed frequent suctioning. I could only slightly move my hips, shoulders, back, quads, and head. None of the movements was strong enough to do anything useful. I couldn't swallow or talk. My decubitus was an open sore. Facially, I could raise my eyebrows, make small expressions, and move my lips to mouth words and form a small smile. I was breathing between 20 and 22 shallow breaths per minute. My weight was 135 lbs. This was my situation as I faced a new staff.

I was in a totally different world now. There was no Rosa, no Theresa, no Norby. Who were my new nurses? What would they be like? I felt abandoned, as if I had been shuttled off to a place where I was out of the way. The place had an ominously cold feeling. The television was off. There were no nurses in sight, no other patients, no sounds—nothing. There was only a heavy silence.

After lying in this frightening stillness for what seemed like hours, the headnurse entered the room.

"Good morning Mr. Sueta. My name is Mrs. Pearce. I know you don't have a call-button to signal for assistance, so I'll have maintenance install one as soon as possible. One of my nurses will be stopping in soon to care for you."

I nodded to let her know I heard what she said. She smiled and left. It was a welcome visit and I was happy to hear I'd have a call-button soon. Her words made me feel a little better.

When a nurse came a little later to suction me and take my vital signs, I thought, "Maybe this ward will be okay."

In the afternoon, my new primary physician, Dr. Glade came to introduce herself. She studied my chart and checked my gag reflex with a tongue depressor. She surprised me by suctioning me. At least she was a doctor who didn't think suctioning patients was "nurse's work." Before she left, she said she would check on me during her daily rounds.

Father Hunkler dropped by to see how I was adjusting to my new surroundings. He stayed a few minutes and said he'd visit often. His pleasant visits were always welcome.

The rest of the day was uneventful. A nurse came to turn me and check my vital signs. When she finished, she turned on the television. It was a welcome diversion from the awful silence. Thankfully, she left the door open and I felt more safe.

I was suctioned and turned every two or three hours, but my insecurity remained. I was all alone in a room without a call-button and no nurses in sight.

The afternoon nurses didn't suction me or turn me as often as the morning shift. A couple of times I had to fight off feelings of panic when I needed suctioning and there was no way to signal for help. At those times, I was on my own and had to control my anxiety and breathing until a nurse finally came by on her rounds.

The first day in my new environment passed slowly. It was a surreal day with my mind in a kind of haze watching every breath, listening to every sound, and staying alert for any sign of trouble. It had been neither a good day nor a bad day.

Alone and without a call-button, my nerves were on edge. I was constantly aware of my vulnerability.

It was sometime after midnight. My room was dark except for the dim light coming from the hallway through the open door. My TV was off. The ward was completely soundless except for the faint echoes of footsteps far down the hall. The silence was eerie.

Suddenly, my room became darker. I turned my head toward the doorway and saw a huge figure blocking the light. The silhouette of a large man loomed in the doorway. With the light behind him, I couldn't see his face.

Whoever he was, I could see he was a patient because he wore pajamas. One thing was certain, he didn't belong in my room. There was something ominous about him. Maybe it was his huge size, maybe it was the slow, ponderous way he moved toward me. What did he want?

My anxiety was building. I knew some patients were not mentally stable. That thought didn't comfort me since I was completely defenseless. In case of trouble, I couldn't yell for help or raise my arms to protect myself.

My imagination took control of my thinking. Irrational thoughts raced through my mind. "What if he tries to hurt me or smother me with a pillow?" In my helpless condition, I wasn't thinking clearly. Any potential threat was magnified out of proportion with reality.

The hulk slowly shuffled up to the side of my bed and stared down at me, not saying a word. Everything was deathly quiet except for the man's heavy breathing. He stood silently, staring down into my face. It was like a nightmare where I was frozen with fear and couldn't run or scream. For many long minutes, neither of us moved.

Then the huge man slowly turned around and shuffled out the door, disappearing as silently as he had come. He was obviously a disoriented patient who had lost the way to his room.

The episode made me acutely aware of how vulnerable I was and how much fear I harbored. Anyone could enter my room and do whatever they wanted. I was defenseless.

It took a while for the tension in my body to ease and allow me to drift off to sleep.

Morning came. To my great relief, a call-button was installed. The button was set next to my cheek so when I turned my head, a light lit in the hallway above my door and on a panel in the nurses' station.

The trach tube in my throat was a foreign object inside my body and the irritation caused extensive, thick fluids to flow, adding to my mucus problem. Whenever I felt mucus was limiting my breathing, I pushed the call-button with my cheek. At first, the nurses responded quickly, but as time passed, they took longer and longer. It was the same problem I had in ICU. The nurses didn't understand that my borderline ability to breathe was affected by even a small amount of mucus. When suctioning produced only a small amount of mucus, once again they believed I was being demanding and manipulative. They began delaying their responses to my call-light.

I signaled for suctioning whenever I felt the need. Was I calling unnecessarily? Was my anxiety over suffocating causing me to overreact and call for suctioning more than I had to? Whether my calls were justified or not could only be proved if I called for help and no one responded at all. Then it could be too late.

Thankfully, most of the nurses were understanding. They could see what my behavior was indirectly telling them about my feelings. They talked to me to assure me everything was okay. It only took a few minutes of their time and actually saved them a lot of trouble because I settled down when I knew they were there if I needed them.

That's all I needed, to be reassured that I was being closely monitored and would be suctioned when I needed it. I just wanted to know the nurses would take care of me and keep me alive. In the hierarchy of human needs, I had the lowest level need—survival.

Mrs. Pearce, the headnurse, saw my anxiety and arranged to have a mental health nurse come and offer counseling to alleviate my fears.

Chapter 16

Managing Is Not Manipulating

"It is a very hard undertaking to seek
to please everybody."
                          Publius Syrus (42 B.C.)

Maryann came the following day. She was an attractive young woman with a warm personality. She had a master's degree in psychiatric nursing and was trained to help patients deal with their anxieties.

During her visit, she used the alphabet board and we "talked" at length. It was a pleasant visit and after she left, I felt we had made a personal connection.

Maryann returned the next day. We talked further and she used acupressure techniques to relax me. The pressure on specific points channeled the energy fields in my body and relieved some of my stress. Maryann saw me almost every day from then on and it didn't take long for us to become good friends.

One day, while Hugh was visiting, I needed suctioning, but all the nurses were busy dealing with more critical patients' needs.

"John, the nurses are all too busy to come right now," Hugh explained.

Using my eyes, I signaled for him to use the vacuum tube hanging on the wall.

He responded with a shocked expression, "I can't do that. I don't know how. I'm sure it's against hospital regulations. I don't want to sound like a wimp, but the sight of mucus makes me feel queasy. I'm sorry, John."

I understood completely. For someone who wasn't a nurse, the sight of thick, greenish secretions could be daunting.

Hugh continued talking with me about other things, but I saw him looking at the suctioning apparatus. He left the room. In a few minutes he returned with a suctioning kit in his hands.

"I asked a nurse if I could get a kit out of the supply room and she said it was okay. I don't know what to do, but I'll give it a try."

Hugh was a mechanical engineer, so I knew he could figure it out.

After carefully reading the instructions on the kit, he opened the envelope, put on the rubber glove, and set up the cleansing solution—just like everyone was supposed to do, but most didn't. He carefully inserted the tube into my trach tube and gently swished it around for about a minute, dipping the tip in the cleansing solution after each withdrawal.

When he was done, my airways felt clear. My old pal had done a good job. All it took was someone who followed the instructions and had a caring attitude.

I smiled to let him know I felt fine. He looked relieved.

I was sure we had broken a few hospital rules, but each time he did it thereafter, Hugh became more skillful.

Since I was in a room by myself, I was allowed to keep the TV on day and night. I needed the sound to help keep me awake. I didn't dare sleep for long periods in case I had a breathing emergency. I slept in short naps during the night and for longer periods of time during the day when more nurses were on duty and more likely to be passing my door if I had an emergency.

One evening, the emergency I feared happened. A small glob of mucus clogged my airway and it became harder to draw a breath. I tried relaxing to see if I was only imagining it, but I wasn't. I labored to breathe for a while, but when I tired and knew I couldn't keep up the effort, I pushed the call-button. My chest muscles were tiring quickly. My air intake was minimal and I could feel my face flushing—the sign my blood oxygen level was low. My chest muscles were almost exhausted when a nursing aide named Castle arrived and suctioned me. Had I been in imminent danger? I'll never know for sure.

Staying alive was a minute by minute fear. The only times I could truly relax was when Virginia, Hugh, or some other person was in the room with me and could summon help if needed. My helplessness kept me in a constant state of dread—irrational or not, it felt just the same to me.

I remembered how in intensive care, I had wished the nurses would leave me alone and not handle me so much. Now I missed all that careful attention and human contact. Hugh and Virginia did many of the little things I needed for my comfort.

Virginia and Bill visited me regularly. They had both reached the 12th step of AA recovery which advocated helping others. Bill visited twice a week, but Virginia came almost every day. She lived nearby and was able to stay for a couple of hours. I looked forward to her visit every afternoon because I never knew which day might be the day I had a breathing emergency. I felt secure with her in the room.

Later, I had another visitor. Virginia had mentioned me to a fellow AA member and he came to visit. Unfortunately, he was still drinking. When he staggered into my room, I saw a man in his thirties, dirty, unshaven, wearing old, wrinkled clothes. He looked and smelled awful.

"Hel...lo." He was so drunk he could barely get the word out. "I'm...Jim." His eyes were all red and tears streamed down his cheeks. He was blubbering like a baby.

I smiled and mouthed hello.

He muttered, "Just...came...to say...hello. Hope...you're okay. Got...to go...now." He staggered out.

Even in that brief encounter, I sensed Jim was a decent type of person. I hoped he would visit me again.

The following day, I had yet another visitor from AA whom Virginia had sent to see me. After introducing himself, Ray said he practiced the laying on of hands and asked if I would like to see if he could help me. I nodded my head.

Ray stood behind my bed and placed the palms of his hands close to my forehead while he spoke soothingly about healing energy flowing into me. I could definitely feel the warmth emanating from his hands. I didn't know if there was an energy flow taking place or if the warmth was simply caused by his nearness. In either case, his presence and the warmth of his hands were relaxing. I welcomed Ray's weekly visits, whether they had a therapeutic effect or not.

The concern and compassion shown by the Alcoholics Anonymous people who visited me was magnificent. I marveled at the selfless way they helped patients in spite of the fact they had such huge problems of their own. They were a wonderful group of people and I highly respected them.

Besides Virginia and Bill's frequent visits, Hugh visited at least twice a week. Father Hunkler also stopped by regularly and there were also volunteer visitors who came to offer good cheer.

One afternoon, I had a very special visit. Rosa and three other nurses from ICU came to see how I was doing and offer me moral support. It was great to see my old friends again. We chatted by using the alphabet board and had a wonderfully warm reunion.

I could tell by their expressions they got a lot of satisfaction from seeing a former patient who was once critically ill, on a ventilator, and totally paralyzed, who was now breathing on his own and able to move many more muscles. My progress validated their nursing efforts.

Until now, I hadn't realized how little positive feedback nurses got and how important it was to them. A lawyer knows how his clients fare, a dentist sees the final results of his work, but nurses seldom see how their patients do after they leave their wards. They see the sickness and suffering and then patients leave before nurses can see the results of all their hard work.

Rosa stayed for a half-hour, but the others had to get back to work. She washed my face, shaved me, and combed my hair. It was a memorable visit from some dedicated nurses.

I knew why the ICU nurses had visited me, but I couldn't figure out why other visitors came. I had nothing to offer them. I couldn't speak and my appearance was often unpleasant with poor grooming and a trach tube stuck in my throat. It was difficult to understand what motivated visitors to keep coming back. Why did they take precious hours out of their own busy lives to spend time with someone in my condition?

I could understand people wanting to visit a pleasant looking patient who could engage them in conversation, or at least thank them for visiting. But, all I could offer were a few facial expressions and brief messages on an alphabet board, if they chose to use it.

Before my illness, I thought my relationships with others was based on impressing them with my appearance and lifestyle. Now I was an unkempt looking patient lying naked under a bedsheet with nothing to offer but my scruffy, voiceless self. All superficiality was stripped away.

Still, my visitors came. They obviously cared about me—but why? What did they get out of it? I wanted to understand what was going on and I had plenty of time to think about it. After days of careful thought, I came to a few conclusions.

I decided my visitors liked me for reasons different than I formerly believed were important. My inability to talk didn't seem to affect my rapport with them. We made a connection regardless. My eyes and facial expressions were able to say what I felt. I was a nonthreatening human being whom they didn't have to try to impress. They could let down their guard and express their own inner selves. They felt free to interact at the most basic, yet deepest, human level.

My helpless condition made them appreciate their own health and realize what was really important in their own lives.

I offered them the opportunity to help someone in need. They could express their humanity by comforting me physically and spiritually. It brought out their best human qualities. Their altruism made them feel good about themselves.

I remembered discussing altruism in a college seminar. The students debated whether altruistic behavior really existed. Most argued that people always behaved selfishly and so-called altruistic deeds were actually done so they would feel good about themselves. Therefore, they concluded every act was selfish.

I challenged them by saying such reasoning begged the question. I argued that doing a kind act with no reward other than an inner feeling of self-satisfaction was the definition of altruism. It was the very essence of altruism. And so it was with my visitors.

Chapter 17

A Change For the Better

"Away from this place of wrath and tears…"
Invictus, William Ernest Henley

On her daily rounds, Dr. Glade always checked my gag reflex with a tongue depressor. She used that as the criterion for whether my condition had improved or not. Her notes read, "Slow gag, no/low voluntary palate elevation."

She was worried that my muscles might be forming contractures and beginning to atrophy, so she called in a group of consulting doctors to check my overall muscle tone. After checking me, they decided that lying immobile was causing my muscles to slowly atrophy. One doctor explained to me what was happening and asked if I wanted steroids to counter-act the deterioration. I knew the dangers of steroids to my liver and other internal organs, so I shook my head "No." As desperately as I wanted to gain muscle strength, I couldn't justify sacrificing my internal health. The price was too high.

Hugh knew how much I hated the room I was in, so during a visit, he asked the headnurse if I could be transferred to a brighter room. Pearce understood and told me she would move me to a room with an outside window. I was excited about moving out of the dark, dreary room.

The very next morning, after all the patients had received their morning care, two nurses packed my belongings and pushed my bed to a room down the hall.

It was a wonderful room! Rather than the depressing room I had been in, this room was bright and cheery and had a big window to the outside. Brilliant sunlight filled the room. I could see the tall buildings nearby in Westwood. I hadn't seen sunlight and the outside world for almost three long months. The sight was overwhelming. Tears streamed down my face. I felt alive again. Why had she put me in that dark, gloomy room with no window to the outside? I guessed it was for the privacy.

The patient in the other bed didn't talk much, but that didn't matter. I wasn't alone. I had another human being near me.

The nurses' station was right outside my door. I wasn't sure that would get me quicker responses, but it was comforting to know nurses were nearby.

My bed faced the window, so all day long I stared at the real world outside while enjoying the warm sunlight. It was a terrific day. I didn't seem to need suctioning as much. Was it because my mind was more relaxed in my new surroundings and my body wasn't tense?

My joy was short-lived. The next day, an unfamiliar nurse came to see me.

She introduced herself with a pleasant, "Good morning Mr. Sueta. My name is Mrs. Redden. I'm from the intermediate care ward. We've been asked to evaluate you to see if you're ready to be transferred to our ward."

I was mentally crushed. I had just been reborn in this wonderful room and now I was being told I had to move to a strange new place with different nurses. My spirits sank.

Mrs. Redden proceeded to check my vital signs and give me an overall check. Making a few notes in her pad, she seemed satisfied and left.

The die was cast. I had no choice in the matter. I would be leaving. Just when things seemed to be getting better, I was on my way to another ward—which might be worse.

To their credit, the rehab nurses did an excellent job on my decubitus. By cleansing it frequently with Betadine, they successfully closed the wound and prevented serious consequences.

I wondered how I would have treated a full-care patient like me if I were a nurse. Nursing was a difficult job with many unpleasant duties that could wear her down. Fortunately, there were those exceptional nurses on the ward who gave me the psychological support I needed to endure. If not for them, my recovery would have been more difficult—if not impossible.

I could understand why some nurses gave their best care to patients who were alert, communicative, and had a good chance for recovery. But, it took an exceptional nurse to compassionately care for very sick patients like me who needed the most help and couldn't express their appreciation. There was little reward for a nurse's hard work with patients like me except for the inner rewards she gave herself and her personal pride in her work. It took an almost saintly attitude to faithfully do all the rigorous nursing duties for patients who seemed chronically ill and had little chance of recovery.

I was leaving. I had no idea what the new ward would be like. All I knew was nurse Redden had called it an intermediate care ward for longterm care patients.

I hoped the new ward would have a staff that was attentive to my suctioning needs and would keep my vital signs stabilized until the myelin sheath covering my motor nerves regenerated—when and if that ever happened. Only time would tell. I was just a helpless patient who was a little pawn being pushed around on a big chessboard. (Though I wasn't happy about moving to an unknown ward, I didn't know that transferring to ward 2-East would turn out to be the best thing that could have happened to me).

The next morning, after all the patients had been fed and medicated, two nurses packed my scant personal belongings and pushed my bed to ward 2-East.

We were met by a nurse who introduced herself as Mrs. Cramer, the headnurse. Though it was all in my file, the rehab nurses told her my medications were 500 units of subcutaneous Heparin b.i.d., 50 mg of Hydrochlorothiazine b.i.d., 20 mg of Potassium b.i.d., 250 mg of Aldomet b.i.d., and 30 cc's of Maalox b.i.d.

Cramer directed the nurses to wheel me into a room with three other patients. They slid me onto my new bed and the rehab nurses left.

Mrs. Cramer was an imposing looking woman, in her late forties I guessed. She was all business.

With only a hint of a smile, she said, "Good morning, Mr. Sweeta, I'm Mrs. Cramer. You'll be on my ward for a while. Your call-button will be working within the hour. Press it whenever you need something and a nurse will help you just as soon as she can."

She spoke perfect English, but I detected a slight accent, possibly Jamaican. That explained her pronunciation of my name, which should be pronounced Su-et'-ah. Her skin color was light though she looked like she was of mixed heritage.

I wasn't sure what to make of her. Was she a friendly, compassionate person or the stern, domineering type? One thing I was sure of, she was in charge. I had no doubts about that. I'd bet she ran the ward with a firm hand.

While she was attending to me, a male nursing aide rushed into the room complaining an older patient was shaking his head and loudly refusing the enema she had ordered, even though he was severely impacted and in pain.

Cramer firmly answered, "Give him the enema." Refusing or not, he got it and that was that.

She had a no-nonsense way about her. That was fine with me. I wanted a headnurse who strictly supervised her nurses.

Before she left, Mrs. Cramer suctioned me and made sure I was comfortable.

Well...here I was, all settled in and wondering how things were going to be. I assessed my condition as I began life on a new ward. My breathing through the trach tube was shallow but adequate. Since it was an irritating foreign object, it caused fluids to develop that needed suctioning every hour or less. Facially, I was able to mouth words, slightly smile, and make small expressions. I could rotate my head, lift my arms a few inches off the bed, minimally move my lower back and hips, and slightly flex my quadriceps. As before, these movements were isolated and didn't allow me to do anything useful. The flexibility in my joints was very limited and getting worse.

The trach tube prevented me from talking, so my only means of communication were the alphabet board and nurses reading my lip movements and facial expressions.

With the television off, the room was quiet. In the bed next to me was the familiar face of Murphy. We were traveling in the same circles. He had been next to me in ICU and I heard him yelling in another room on the rehab ward. That meant he had had his trach tube removed and could talk. Speaking gave him a tremendous advantage that I didn't have. It was the ultimate tool for communicating with the staff. Speaking made you a person, not just an unknown lump of flesh and bones. It meant the nurses could know your personality and relate to you. There was so much I wanted to say, but my inner self was bottled up inside my voiceless body.

I felt as vulnerable as only a paralyzed, voiceless person could feel. Everything around me was unfamiliar. Not being able to speak and express my needs and feelings kept my anxiety level high. I lay in bed, listening to every sound, waiting to see how long it would be before I needed suctioning and how quickly a nurse responded.

The first days on the new ward were tolerable. I still needed frequent suctioning, but it was done quickly enough to keep my anxiety in check. Mrs. Cramer had the ward well organized so I had no major problems with the staff. The nurses did their best to take care of my many needs and were hard working, well disciplined and I received good basic care.

Thankfully, bedbathing was done in the morning. During bedbaths, I had conflicting thoughts. I was a normal man, so having a female nurse wash my groin area with warm water was a pleasurable experience. I had to use a lot of mental discipline to walk the fine line between enjoying the sexual sensations while simultaneously diverting my thoughts to avoid the obvious reaction. I didn't always succeed.

I rarely had the same nurse two days in a row, so only a few nurses became familiar with my care. Nurse Shirley Redden took the time to become fairly well acquainted. Shirley was one of those nurses who had left nursing for a few years and returned after she had had a chance to take a long break from the rigors of nursing and come back with a fresh outlook. The time off worked well and she was once again enjoying nursing. It seemed nurses all needed to step back at times and see things from a fresh perspective.

A nurse on the afternoon shift made a special effort to become acquainted with me. Mrs. Desdemona Agard was an older, black lady who was wonderfully compassionate and had a delightful, girlish laugh. She was a highly experienced nurse who had learned her craft in the hellholes of Guyana where she had practiced nursing with scant supplies and under extreme conditions.

Mrs. Agard was unbelievably kind. She did whatever she could to make my life more pleasant. She suctioned me whenever I asked. I felt so secure under her watchful eye that I didn't seem to generate as much fluid and required less suctioning when she was assigned to me. She was an outstanding nurse—a nurse's nurse.

Using the alphabet board, I told Mona I missed being able to hold a book and turn pages so I could read. In response, she brought books from home and read classic poetry and passages from inspirational books like Gibran's The Prophet. I looked forward to her afternoon readings.

However, none of the other nurses cared for me on a regular basis and had the opportunity to know me personally.

Life on the ward followed an organized sameness and the days seemed to run together in a big blur. Weeks passed quickly and before I knew it, December rolled around. I had been on the ward for three months with no major changes in my paralysis.

Christmas arrived quietly. I didn't know why, but I had no visitors during the holidays. Except for the Salvation Army band and their volunteer well-wishers, no one came—neither family nor friends. Hugh was probably busy with the holiday activities of his family. Virginia too. I hadn't seen Charlene and Chris for months. Being alone in a hospital during the holidays was worse than at any other time. Christmas had always been a special time for me so I felt the loneliness more deeply.

The only outside visitor I had during the holidays was Charlie Holmes, a hospital volunteer. Charlie was a wonderful guy, always smiling, always a gentleman. He was affectionately known as "the music man" because he came to the wards and played records on an old phonograph and accompanied the music on a large double-bass he called Suzie.

Charlie made the rounds of the different wards, one day on this ward, the next day on another. He'd arrive in the afternoon, pushing the small cart that held his equipment. He would set up his phonograph in the hallway, dust off his precious collection of old vinyl records, and start playing. Charlie had been playing on the wards for ten years, meticulously rotating his library of golden oldies.

Charlie was a retired, disabled veteran who had decided to devote his free time to entertaining hospitalized veterans. He was a passable musician, but he liked to be thought of as a person whose goal was to break up the drudgery of hospital life and used his music as a vehicle for getting patients together to talk, share stories, and forget their suffering for a little while. When patients heard Charlie's music, they came out of their rooms to chat with him and with each other. That's exactly what he wanted. Bedridden patients listened to the old, familiar tunes from their beds and nostalgicized. There were times when no patients came out in the hall to see him. That didn't bother Charlie. He played his music in the empty hallway anyway, knowing patients were listening in their rooms. Nurses enjoyed the music too as they hummed along while caring for patients.

Charlie's music and friendly conversation helped me get through the holidays. It transported my thoughts to Christmas times in the past when things were better. Christmas came and went quietly.

The week after Christmas passed quickly too and a new year was beginning. Would this be the year my paralysis reversed itself and I returned to normal living? I hoped so. Until that time, I resigned myself to simply getting by one day at a time.

The hospital routine dragged on. January turned into February, then March. I was receiving good nursing care and suctioning was done often enough to calm my nerves.

In an effort to enable me to speak, my doctor tried a cuffless, fenestrated tube. The tube had holes in it and allowed exhaled air to pass from my lungs upward through my larynx. Unfortunately, it didn't work.

Dr. Bruce from speech therapy brought a Cooper-Rand laryngeal tone generator to substitute for my vocal cords. That failed too.

I was shifted back to a cuffed tube, but I couldn't figure out why I still had a trach tube in my throat after getting off the ventilator. If I could breath on my own, what was the function of the trach tube? I thought it was kept in because it made suctioning easier.

One afternoon, while Maryann was doing acupressure, I felt my cuff needed inflation. I mouthed the problem and she dutifully pumped air into it. Cramer was standing nearby and decided to call an otolaryngologist to check on whether I needed a new tube.

Dr. Abemayor arrived within a few minutes. He was troubled when he saw I was breathing on my own and still had a trach tube in my throat. Checking my chart, he saw I had been off the ventilator for six months.

He asked firmly, "Why does this patient still have his trach tube?"

Cramer and Maryann answered they didn't know.

Dr. Abemayor said, "I'm going to remove it. It should have been out a long time ago."

I had a terrible feeling of dread. Even though I suspected it should have been removed months ago, that tube in my throat was my lifeline. I breathed through it. It represented life itself to me. No one was going to remove it if I could prevent it— neither an ENT doctor nor anyone else. I shook my head, protesting I didn't want it removed. Maryann felt my anxiety and asked the doctor to leave it in.

Dr. Abemayor was a young doctor, but he had a confidence about him that was unmistakable. He had no doubts that the tube should come out and was unwavering in his decision.

I was frightened. If he removed the tube, would I be able to breathe through the hole in my throat? If it closed, would I be able to sufficiently breathe through my nose and mouth? I was confused and alarmed.

In spite of my tremendous fear, I was rational enough to recognize that Dr. Abemayor knew what he was doing. I felt the power of his self-confidence. If he was so damned sure the tube should come out, I decided to trust him. I nodded my agreement. Let's do it.

Dr. Abemayor untied the string around my neck that held the tube in place and pulled out the tube. Everyone stood by and watched my breathing. Cramer and Maryann waited in anticipation along with me.

A minute passed. Two minutes. After ten minutes had passed, it was clear to everyone that I was breathing adequately through my nose, mouth, and partially closed hole in my throat. The tube was thrown away. (The removal of the trach tube was the beginning of a dramatic improvement in my progress! Dr. Abemayor's decision would change everything).

I began to slowly unwind as I realized I was breathing okay. After a year, I was finally free of the tracheostomy. No more unpleasant tube changes, no more leaky cuffs, and most important, no more suctioning of mucus caused by a foreign object in my body.

I couldn't help wondering whether the trach tube would have been removed earlier if an ENT doctor had been brought in to evaluate me. The overly long presence of the tube could have caused necrosis of the mucosa and tracheal cartilage.

Something else resulted from the removal of the trach tube with its balloon seal. I could speak in a whispered tone. Some of my exhaled air was now passing through the partially open hole in my throat, but some was passing over my now open vocal cords. In a whispering way, I could talk!

My silent world was about to change. I began talking in a whisper with the nurses, my visitors, and anyone else who would listen. After a year of silence, I had a lot of things to say. My inner self was eager to be set free from the bonds of silence. The staff would soon be able to know the real me, both good and bad.

Chapter 18

Primary Nursing and the Turnaround

"A guardian angel o'er his life presiding ..."
Samuel Mayor (1763-1855)

I was amazed at how much my relationships with nurses changed after I could talk. There was a dramatic difference between the way some nurses treated me before I could speak and how the same nurses treated me afterwards. For some, it was as if I had been a nonperson and now I was a real human being. Once they could talk with me, their nursing went from a quiet, businesslike way of taking care of me to an animated, friendly manner that wanted to interact on a personal level.

In a similar way, I had a different attitude toward nurses after I could speak with them and know them personally. Some nurses I previously thought were cold and aloof, I now saw as friendly and compassionate.

I humbly remembered those outstanding nurses on the previous wards who had taken the time to communicate with me using the alphabet board and by reading my facial expressions before I could speak. They gave me a chance to express emotions that were bottled up inside me. They were willing to form a bond with me at a time when I needed their compassion the most and probably deserved it the least. I wished more nurses understood how important it was to connect with patients who appeared to be mentally unaware, but were actually alert and anxious to communicate. Those caring nurses who had made a connection with me during those difficult times were what made my life bearable.

The alphabet board was thrown away. I could now express myself without it. It was a whole new way of interacting.

However, the ability to speak was a mixed blessing. It meant I could have pleasant conversations with nurses, but it also meant I could express my feelings when I disagreed with them.

I still needed help to get out of bed, toilet, dress, brush my teeth, and so many other things. Not being able to do the simplest things for myself was incredibly frustrating. I wished I could spend one whole day without asking a nurse for help.

Cramer had assigned herself to me that day. As headnurse, she didn't have to do bedside care, but she chose to be hands-on involved with the patients. I was having a bad day and was surly as she bedbathed me and changed my sheets. Cramer didn't let my bad mood bother her and ignored my irritability.

Nevertheless, I realized I was being difficult and felt guilty, so I said to her, "Try to bear with me, Mrs. Cramer."

My plea for understanding touched a responsive chord within her and prompted her to answer, "Mr. Sweeta, I've been giving a lot of thought to your situation and I've decided to be your primary nurse. I'll be your nurse everyday. On other shifts and whenever I'm not on duty, I will assign one other nurse to care for you under my instructions. You'll have the same nurses everyday. We'll get to know you better and you'll get to know us. There will be consistency in your care. I believe you have the potential to improve more than you have been and I intend to help you."

My eyes welled up with tears and I couldn't speak. I wasn't sure why Cramer had made this unexpected decision, but I didn't care why. The only thing that mattered was I knew I would receive the best nursing care possible. I didn't know it at the time, but she had made a decision that would totally change my recovery.

Until that day, I had been receiving team nursing. I never knew which nurse would be assigned to me for the day. It was confusing and disruptive. With the same nurses everyday, I could relax because I knew what to expect during every shift of every day. Instead of general care, I'd receive individualized care. I would have a consistent routine.

The assigned nurses could also get into a routine. They would be patient-centered, not task-centered. They could relate to me as a person because they would get to know me as a person, not just "bed 55." They would be giving holistic care and could take personal pride in my progress because they would be directly involved in it. Of course, the reverse was also true. It meant they each had a responsibility and were accountable. If I had a problem, their care was directly open to criticism because they were the only nurses involved.

I remembered that my mother had had a primary nurse assigned to her when she was in the hospital decades earlier and it worked out well. That must have been the way hospitals used to be. I wondered why they had changed. Patients had a primary doctor, so why not a primary nurse?

But, the real prize for me was that I would have, not just any nurse, but a highly qualified one as my primary nurse.

That afternoon, I found out that Cramer had assigned Mrs. Agard as my nurse on the afternoon shift. How lucky could I get?

As a crowning touch, in Cramer's absence, another old pro named Mrs. Hunt would fill in. She was a wonderful black lady who had earned a masters degree in nursing and had once been a consultant to hospitals in Western Africa. After work, she took care of her invalid mother, so she understood my needs.

Her warm smile and genuine sincerity endeared her as a friend to everyone. I never heard Mrs. Hunt speak an unkind word about anyone, nor they of her. She was liked by all.

The night shift nurse wasn't as important since no care was given during sleeping hours. Bedbaths were done in the morning. I wished ICU had also bathed me in the mornings and not subjected me to the middle of the night ordeal.

Even at this early stage of my recovery, I recognized the importance of having Cramer, Agard, and Hunt taking care of me. Between them, they had over ninety years of the most highly skilled nursing experience possible. If nurses were "angels of mercy," I had three of them.   It was a new beginning.

The hole in my throat continued to slowly close by itself, without the need for suturing. The more it closed, the better I could speak because more air was passing over my vocal cords. Though I was breathing fairly well now, Cramer noticed my nostrils were clogged. She sat down next to my bed and took a tweezers to very carefully remove what turned out to be a mass of dried mucus that had accumulated during the past twelve months. After she finished, my airways were fully open and the improved airflow made a tremendous difference in my breathing.

That evening at dinnertime, Mrs. Agard tested my ability to swallow by placing a small spoonful of orange sherbet on my tongue. My taste buds had not experienced food for a year. When the orange sherbet touched my tongue, it created a taste explosion in my mouth. The taste was magnified a hundred times as my taste buds sprang to life after months of dormancy. It was incredibly delicious.

I easily swallowed the sherbet. Despite the long inactivity, my throat muscles were also responding. Agard proceeded to spoonfeed me applesauce and soft vegetables. I swallowed them with no problem. The flavors were glorious. I was eating— really eating!

The very next day the NG tube and liquid foodbag were removed and I began receiving a foodtray with a special diet. In only a few days, I was eating regular food, three meals a day. Eating real food again was an unbelievable pleasure— psychologically as well as physically. I savored every bite and ate everything on my tray.

One day while Mrs. Agard was patiently feeding me one small spoonful at a time, I began to choke. A piece of food had gotten stuck in my throat and I couldn't cough hard enough to dislodge it. She immediately began slapping me on the back to clear it. After a few slaps, the obstruction popped out. It turned out to be a small piece of meat, no bigger than a pea, that had caused my epiglottis to malfunction and close off my trachea. Once again, I was reminded of how small an obstruction it took to interfere with breathing. I swallowed more carefully after that.

I now had two of the three things I wanted the most when I was in intensive care. I remembered telling myself in ICU that all I would ever want was to breathe without a ventilator, to eat real food, and to walk. Walking would have to wait until I was stronger.

I had thought that once I could do those three things, anything else would be unimportant. But, now I thought differently. I wanted more. Besides walking, I wanted to use my hands to dress myself, feed myself, exercise, and do whatever else it took to get back to the real world. I needed new goals. I needed something new to hope and strive for—

otherwise, I'd stagnate mentally and physically. I had to move on to the next level.

Mrs. Cramer not only tended to my physical well-being, she kept in touch with my mental well-being. In the afternoons after all the patients had been cared for, she came to my room and we had long talks about my progress, my goals, and life in general.

Through our conversations, I got to know Mrs. Cramer well. I learned she had been born in Jamaica and was still a Jamaican at heart, with a lot of pride in her heritage. I enjoyed listening to her lilting Jamaican accent. Trained by British doctors, she spoke perfect English—except when she wanted to make a point. Then she slipped into a heavy Jamaican accent to quote some wise old saying.

In Jamaica, she had been a public health nurse for twenty-five years. She had worked alone in out-of-the-way places, driving down dusty backroads in her little car. In the countryside, she tended to mostly poor people who received little other medical attention. Cramer did whatever needed to be done with whatever supplies she had or could improvise. She inoculated thousands of people, tended wounds, delivered babies, and gave preventive medical care. Her incredibly broad range of nursing skills was learned the hard way, in the field all by herself. Through her broad experiences, Cramer had developed a practical knowledge of nursing that would prove invaluable to me.

This was the nurse who took me into her personal care and decided to be my primary nurse. I would be the recipient of all the knowledge she gleaned from years of intensive nursing.

As headnurse, she was prim and formal. She never used first names for patients or staff. She never called me John. Neither staff nor visitors were allowed to sit on the beds or eat off patients' trays. Hospital rules were followed exactly, with no exceptions.

In the mornings, even before I saw her, I could hear her coming down the hall as she went from door to door, saying "Good morning" with a Jamaican lilt to each patient. Once you heard her voice, you knew everything was going to be okay. She was in charge and the ward would function smoothly. It was amazing how comforted patients felt when they had confidence in the headnurse. They truly believed they would be safe and well cared for as long as she was in charge.

Cramer was an independent woman long before women's lib came along. She was a combination of logic and gut instincts. Her ways were clear and simple. She balanced toughness with sensitivity. However, she hated being called "tough," preferring "strong." Underneath she could be sensitive and almost fragile. Little things touched her. Many times I saw tears well up in her eyes when we discussed her children or some past nursing incident that touched her deeply. She still fondly remembered a man in Jamaica who cut open a fresh coconut to quench her thirst after her long, dusty trip to care for his wife.

Cramer's primary nursing care coupled with Dr. Abemayor's removal of my trach tube was the start of my turnaround. But, my problems were far from over. I was starting my recovery with no motor skills. Each small step of progress was a hard fought battle. Every setback was distressing. My agonizingly slow progress was extremely disappointing and the inner battle continued.

Cramer asked me if I'd like to move into the private room next door. She thought I'd get more rest without the commotion of three other patients. I wasn't sure I wanted to be in a room by myself, but I agreed. The new room was sunlit by a large window that overlooked the first floor's rooftop patio. I was satisfied with the room and happy with her decision to move me.

The first step of my rehabilitation was to start using the commode instead of the bedpan. She lifted me out of bed with a Hoyer Lift, transferred me into my wheelchair and then the commode. Cramer knew patients eliminated better in a sitting position rather than lying down. She compared it to some women in Jamaica who gave birth easier in a birthing chair rather than lying down in bed. The change worked well for me. From then on, I was lifted out of bed every morning for toileting and then put in my wheelchair to sit for a few hours.

Cramer's next move was to start my physical therapy. She had a nursing aide named Mrs. Wilson wheel me to the hydro-therapy room every morning.

Hydrotherapy wasn't a pleasant experience. Being lowered in a sling into moderately warm water was uncomfortable and frightening. I had an instinctive fear of drowning since I had no way to keep afloat if something went wrong. I was lying helplessly on my back with water up to my lower neck that might get into my throat-hole, nose, and then my lungs .

In the hydrotherapy tub, the water's buoyancy allowed me to move muscles I couldn't move otherwise. In the beginning, I could only wiggle my arms and legs, but in the following weeks, I was able to move more broadly and build some strength.

Wheeling me around everyday gave my wheelchair pusher, aide Wilson, a chance to talk to me about her problems. She was anxious to tell someone about her problems and I was a captive audience. Every day, I heard about how tired she was and I listened to stories about her headaches, backaches, and sore feet. She complained so much, I wondered if we shouldn't trade places. I didn't mind her telling me about her aches and pains, but not every day. I had my own aches and pains.

Going to hydrotherapy and other activities made the days pass faster. I was a busy guy. I was Hoyer lifted out of bed every day for toileting, eating, and then on to hydrotherapy, and sunbathing on the patio.

Sitting in my wheelchair felt all right for the first few hours, but in the afternoon I became uncomfortable. My buttocks and back usually became sore and I wanted to lie down. Getting back in bed always felt so-o-o good. I could relax between the nice, cool sheets and settle down to watch the afternoon and evening TV shows. It was one of my few pleasures.

At around three o'clock, I usually asked Cramer to put me back in bed. However, she always made me stay up a while longer by saying, "Not now, Mr. Sweeta. I'm busy and all the nurses are helping other patients, so you'll have to sit there one more hour." It was always the same answer, no matter what time I asked her.

Of course, I knew what she was doing. She wanted me to get used to sitting up for longer and longer periods of time until I could sit up all day. No matter how good her intentions were, it didn't help my sore gluteus maximus.

As a result, I figured out a way to outfox the fox. About an hour before I was really ready, I asked to be put back in bed. Naturally, she told me, "One more hour, Mr. Sweeta." Then, like clockwork, one hour later, she always came and put me back in bed. It was just what I wanted. She thought she was fooling me by keeping me up an extra hour, but she didn't realize she was doing exactly what I wanted. She was satisfied and so was I. It took some Hollywood acting on my part because Cramer knew most of the tricks patients play. It was fun matching wits with her.

I couldn't let the fox win *all* the time.

On Sundays, Cramer had Mrs.Wilson wheel me to the hospital chapel for services. It was relaxing to sit in serene surroundings, away from the hustle and bustle of the ward. Attending Sunday services were other patients, hospital staff, and many well-dressed visitors.The smell of fresh flowers, soft organ music, and inspirational sermons from Father Hunkler made the services something I looked forward to.

Cramer wanted me to take advantage of as many activities and therapies as I could, so she added occupational therapy to my already busy schedule. I spent mornings in hydrotherapy and afternoons in occupational therapy. It was a pleasant experience because there were no difficult physical demands and I got a chance to talk to other patients and therapists.

I was assigned to a nice therapist named Judy, a lady in her late forties I guessed. She focused on trying to increase the range of motion in my hands. My knuckle joints were frozen solid with adhesions because my hands had lain open, palms down, on the bed beside me for a whole year. After such a long time of nonflexing, the knuckle joints had formed fibrous tissue and my hands were stuck in an open position. In addition, the muscles in my forearms had atrophied and I had no strength to even try closing my hands.

Through the following weeks, Judy carefully bent my finger joints as much as she could, but the fibrous tissue would not break loose because the tendons had severely contracted and wouldn't stretch enough for me to make a fist. I suspected my hands had passed the point of no return.

I had played the piano since I was eight years old and had even played professionally. The joints of my once nimble fingers were now frozen in an open position. I doubted if I would ever again be able to express myself through my music and feel the exhilaration of playing the songs I loved. I'd miss playing more than I dared think about. It was another discouraging loss to add to all my other losses.

One morning, while Cramer was finishing my morning care, Mrs. Wilson came into the room. She looked troubled as she told Cramer she had a problem and wanted to discuss it privately. I remembered how Mrs. Wilson had unloaded a list of her aches and pains on me.

Instead of responding, "Let's go to my office and talk," Cramer changed the subject. She reminded Wilson of her assignments for the day and terminated the conversation.

I said to Cramer, "Don't you think you should have listened to her?" But, knowing she usually had good reasons for her actions, I held back. I wanted to hear her reasoning. I remembered reading studies that showed managers who got too involved with their employees' personal problems, made bad managers. They got so bogged down in their employees' troubles that they weren't taking care of their managerial duties.

Cramer said, "I don't want to reinforce complaining. Not responding accomplishes three things. First, the problems are not magnified by dwelling on them. Secondly, the patients are better cared for without nursing time lost in long discussions. And most important, it is good for the nurse to concentrate on her duties instead of herself. She actually gets a mental break because it takes her mind off her own problems. They may resent it at the time, but in the long run, they are grateful because helping others is the best way to forget about yourself and the work becomes therapeutic."

I asked, "But, doesn't that make some nurses dislike you?"

She answered, "It does for a while, but in time they respect me for keeping them focused and organized. You can't respect someone without liking them. In time, they do both."

I had to think about that one.

She continued, "If a nurse is troubled to the point she can't perform her duties and is clearly overstressed, I work with her and offer suggestions to help her. If necessary, I make an appointment with psychiatric services to get her counseling. However, if the problems are just the usual complaining and don't warrant counseling or therapy, like Mrs. Wilson's, my general rule is, 'Leave your problems at the door.' "

She concluded, "Did you notice Mrs. Wilson went right back to work without a fuss?"

One person who never complained was Mrs. Martin, the wife of a patient in the next room. Mrs. Martin was a woman in her forties whose bedridden husband had an irreversible form of paralysis that was slowly progressing. The prognosis was he would continually decline till his breathing stopped. He was a "no code."

Mrs. Martin came to the hospital every day at 7 AM and stayed till after dinnertime. She had done this seven days a week for the past five years, only missing one day in all that time—for which she felt so guilty, she vowed never to miss another one. She was the epitome of a devoted wife.

Mrs. Martin did complete care for her husband. She toileted him in bed, gave him bedbaths, total grooming, and fed him three meals a day, one spoonful at a time. It was an incredible example of love and devotion. The nurses only had to give him medications and monitor his vital signs. She did all the rest.

Despite her rough situation, Mrs. Martin had a wonderful sense of humor. She was a lot of fun and we enjoyed joking with each other.

One afternoon I asked her how late the hospital store stayed open, so I could have someone buy me some toothpaste. She said she didn't know but she'd find out. I waited anxiously for her to return and tell me how much time I had before the store closed.

Hours later, she came into my room and said, "You know that question you asked me this morning?"

I responded impatiently, "Yes, yes, what's the answer?'

She said, "I forgot the question."

I just shook my head and rolled my eyes. She was a gem.

Mrs. Martin's primary care of her husband paid off in his physical and mental well-being just as Cramer's primary care was paying dividends for me. Now that I was eating regular food, I had put on eight pounds of healthy muscle. My weight had increased to 153 pounds.

Before my illness, I used to drink a beer once a day, so I asked my doctor if he'd approve my having a bottle of beer every afternoon. I told him it would relax me and help me gain weight. He saw nothing wrong with the idea and wrote his authorization. Cramer was kind enough to bring in the beer and kept it in the refrigerator. Every afternoon was "Miller time."

Another patient also had his afternoon pick-me-up. Mr. Calibri was a delightful fellow, ninety-six years young. Every afternoon when Cramer brought me my bottle of Millers, she brought Mr. Calibri his daily shot of brandy—prescribed by his doctor of course. I think that helped keep the old gent sprightly.

His thin face had a perpetual smile on it and he never complained even when he was in pain. He just kept smiling. Sometimes he spoke clearly, sometimes he was hard to understand. If you simply listened to his muttering and smiled as if you understood, that was fine. All he wanted was a little attention.

In spite of his age, he liked to be out of bed and amongst people. He'd sit in his wheelchair in the hallway from breakfast to dinnertime, saying "hello" to everyone who passed by. He called the ward "home." On Sunday mornings, he regularly went to mass to receive Holy Communion.

He was a wiry old Italian who still had an eye for the ladies, despite his age. In fact, the nurses had to be watchful around him. He liked to hold hands with any nurse who stopped to talk with him. One nurse let him kiss her on the cheek whenever she tended to him. One day I saw him touch a nurse's leg as he told her how pretty she was. She got a kick out of it and laughed as she politely brushed his hand away. Old Mr.Calibri never stopped flirting.

It was nice to have him on the ward because he made everyone smile when they saw him with that funny little woolen hat he always wore to keep his head warm. It made him look like Jacques Cousteau.

In contrast to Mr. Calibri's zest for life, was another old man that I met in the hallway. He was sitting in a wheelchair next to mine. After we introduced ourselves, Mr. Rab told me he had had a stroke that left him paralyzed on one side. He was eighty-five years old and he candidly said he was tired of the daily struggle of living. He became angry when I jokingly suggested he might make it to a hundred. I hadn't realized he was serious about not wanting to live any longer. Like the song said, "He was tired a livin, but scared a dyin."

Even at his advanced age, Mr. Rab's mind was still clear. He told me his friends were all dead and he never saw his children who lived far away in New York. That was the difference between him and Mr. Calibri who had a large support group of loving family and friends who visited him often. Mr. Rab felt the few moments of pleasure he had during each lonely day weren't worth all the pain.

It saddened me to listen to this cheerless, old gentleman who felt there was no point in living any longer. He had reached a point where he felt his life had no purpose. Nobody cared, so why should he?

It was dinnertime and I had to leave Mr. Rab to his forlorn thoughts. The episode made me realize how important a caring family and support people were to a patient's well-being. For some patients, the support of others was the difference between wanting to live and wanting to die.

Chapter 19

Physical and Psychological Progress

"Every joy is gain,
And gain is gain, however small."
Robert Browning (1812-1889)

In the afternoon, I kept my OT appointment. Judy continued working on my hands and fingers. She was aware I could move my arms a little, so she had an idea. She asked me if I would like an electric wheelchair, explaining it would have a joystick that I could push with my palm and didn't require using my fingers. It would allow me to have the freedom to go wherever I wanted in the hospital without needing someone to push me.

It was a no-brainer. I told her I'd love to have one and to order it as soon as possible.

The electric wheelchair arrived from the hospital's storage room in two days. With a few basic instructions from Judy, operating it was simple. I had a new independence. Now I could take myself to my therapy sessions and explore the hospital instead of being confined to the ward all day or depending on Wilson to push me. For the next week, I cruised all over the hospital, exploring the huge building inside and out. The feeling of freedom was incredibly liberating.

My movements in the hydrotherapy tub had improved enough for the hydrotherapist to recommend moving my therapy into the gym next door where I could receive more extensive exercise. He made the arrangement on the phone.

The next morning, I piloted my electric wheelchair into the gym and identified myself. A young fellow named Rick came over and introduced himself as my physical therapist. Once again, I lucked out. There were eight therapists in the gym. Four were women, two were older men, and two were young men. Patients requiring less lifting and moving could be helped by the women and older PTs, but in my condition, I needed a strong young man. Lifting me required a man's strength. That was a simple fact. A woman or older man would not have risked straining their backs and would have avoided lifting me entirely. Rick was in his late twenties and athletic. He was just what I needed to lift me out of the wheelchair and onto the therapy bench for range of motion. I had no arm or leg strength to help him stand me up and transfer, so he had to support my full, limp weight by himself.

After a few days of range of motion exercises lying on the bench, Rick decided to try me on the tilt table. I was strapped down and the table was rotated to an upright position. Standing was a whole new experience. I hadn't been upright in over a year. It felt great to be in a standing position. It put my internal organs in a normal position and allowed proper blood circulation. Surprisingly, I wasn't dizzy. Rick thought the change in blood flow might make me lightheaded, but it didn't. Instead of looking up at people from a sitting or lying position, I was now looking at them eye to eye. I was even looking down at those shorter than my six-foot height. Lying down was a helpless feeling, but standing gave me a sense of power and equality. It was another milestone.

After two weeks of standing in the tilt table with no dizziness or other problems, I suggested to Rick that I wanted to try standing between the parallel bars. He was all for it. First, he strapped a full leg brace on my weaker left leg to keep the knee from buckling. Then, Rick placed his hands in my armpits and stood me up. It took all his strength to get me up because my arms and legs had almost no strength to assist him. While balancing me, he let me stand on my own two feet for a minute.

During the next two weeks, the length of standing time was gradually increased. Once I was fairly stable standing, Rick had me try a few steps between the parallel bars. With his support and whatever arm and leg strength I had, I managed a few shuffling steps. It wasn't much, but it was a start.

I was emotionally high. I wanted to hurry back to the ward to tell Cramer I had "walked." Excitement was pouring out of me and I needed to share it with someone.

Back on the ward, I excitedly said, "Mrs. Cramer, I took my first steps. I walked!"

With no show of emotion, she replied, "That's good. Tomorrow you'll do better."

With Cramer, there was no resting on your laurels, you had to keep pushing forward and never be satisfied. Actually, I was surprised she even said, "That's good."

From then on, progress in the parallel bars was slow but steady. It required heavy exertion from both Rick and me.

As I struggled to walk in the parallel bars while wearing the huge leg brace, I thought about the people outside the hospital who didn't appreciate their good health. Here I was, fighting through incredible frustration and pain, trying to improve my physical movements by fractions of an inch, while outside the hospital were thousands of thrill seekers who didn't appreciate their healthy bodies and were willing to cripple themselves for a cheap thrill.

I had no sympathy for extreme sports thrill seekers who sacrificed their bodies for an adrenalin rush. They didn't realize what they had and risked it all for a temporary high. Sky divers, bungee jumpers, BASE jumpers, rock climbers, extreme skiers, and all those other idiots who had no understanding of what it was like to lose their ability to walk, feed themselves, and do the thousands of things it was necessary to do in everyday life. If they understood how blessed they were to have sound, healthy bodies, they might get their adrenalin rush in less insane ways.

When I finished my parallel bar walking, I sat back in my wheelchair and reflected on what fools these mortals be. I was exhausted and hurting. My leg throbbed with pain as Rick removed the heavy leg brace. I was going through hell just to achieve the slightest gain.

In a week, with great effort and Rick's help, I was able to walk the length of the parallel bars. In the following week, I managed to improve and felt I didn't need the heavy leg brace anymore, so I asked Rick not to put it on.

When I told Cramer about my progress, she said, "Walk good mon." She explained that was a Jamaican saying to wish someone good luck. It seemed to fit my situation.

Things were going well in the gym, but I wasn't satisfied. Though I was making progress, it was slow and painful. I had been in the hospital for a year and a half with no end in sight. Meanwhile, outside the hospital everything I had worked for was gone. All my real estate had been sold because I couldn't make the mortgage payments. They were sold at ridiculously low prices and I received very little profit from them. My Cadillac had been totaled by a hit-and-run driver while parked on the street. My son Chris was failing in highschool. It seemed everything had gone downhill and I was totally helpless to do anything about it. My former life had fallen apart and my future was a big question mark. The frustration was burning a hole in me.

I couldn't help feeling down—way down. I skipped my physical therapy appointment. I couldn't stop thinking, "What's the use? I don't need all this pain and frustration. Everything I worked so hard for is gone. I just want to be left alone."

There was a perverse pleasure in feeling sorry for myself. A part of my mind seemed to enjoy the self-pity. My masochistic side liked playing the part of an unfortunate victim of life.

After hours of depressing thoughts, I became aware that I was being overly dramatic. Thoughts such as "What's the use?" "I can't go on," and "How much can a man take?" reminded me of lines I'd heard in movies. Once I was conscious of my Hollywood dramatics, I stopped my self-indulgence. I knew that what I was doing wasn't helping me.

It would have been so easy to stay in my room, feel sorry for myself, and watch TV all day. However, I knew I had to get busy and stop moping around. I really didn't feel like it, but the rational part of my mind seemed to be compelling me to head in the direction of the gym. Every two minutes, I thought about turning my wheelchair around, but for some reason I kept going.

Once I got to the gym, I felt a little better. Everyone was busy, so I decided to try exercising on my own. I started out slowly by walking a length in the parallel bars. It went well. My blood was starting to pump faster throughout my body and my brain was clearing.

Rick saw me and came over to chat while I continued exercising. I spied Murphy and rolled over to his wheelchair to ask him how he was doing. He proudly showed me the new movements he had in his arms and legs.

It felt good to focus on things and people outside myself. My dark mood was slowly fading. Without a lot of psychological self-analysis, I had taken control of my mind by taking control of my body. I found it was impossible for me to think negatively while my body was busy exercising and my mind was focused on others.

By the time I finished exercising and chatting, I felt much better. My muscles were pleasantly tired and I was in a positive mood. It amazed me how easily my mind was able to shift from negative to positive thoughts simply by plunging myself into physical and mental activity instead of sitting around and letting my mind feed on itself. My bad mood was completely gone and I felt fine as I returned to my room.

Mrs. Hunt stopped in and said she had something for me. She knew I liked music from the operettas, so she had taped recordings of Showboat and Carousel for me to play on my tape player. She said she'd be back later to read to me from a book of poetry she just bought. Mrs. Hunt was a caring person as well as a fine nurse and wanted to make sure my mind was stimulated as well as my body.

I was feeling too good to just sit there on the ward, so I drove to a grassy area near a flower garden and parked my wheelchair. It was quiet there, with only muted sounds of traffic far off in the distance. The evening was pleasantly cool and the air had the fragrant smell of flowers in bloom and freshly cut grass. The sprinklers had been on a short while ago, so everything smelled pure and clean.

I leaned back in my wheelchair as I breathed in the cool night air and looked up at the sky. It was a clear summer night with millions of sparkling stars. The evening was peaceful and quiet. It amazed me how our little planet could travel through the sky without harm because of the vastness of space.

The size of the universe staggered my imagination. Did it have boundaries or was the universe like a moebius that curled back upon itself and had no beginning or end? Trying to figure it all out with my puny mind was fun, but fruitless.

After a pleasant hour, I returned to my room and thought about how insignificant me and my problems actually were....

Chapter 20

The Meaning of "Handicapped"

"I believe there are a number of questions
that it is no use our asking, because
they can never be answered."
                                    Julian Huxley

Returning from occupational therapy one afternoon, I zipped past the nurses' station at my wheelchair's full speed. Cramer followed me into my room.

"Mr. Sweeta, I know you like using that electric wheelchair because it's easy and fun, but I would prefer you go back to using a regular wheelchair. I want you to use your arms to develop strength and not be sitting back letting the chair do all the work."

I was enjoying the wheelchair and replied, "What if I don't want to," I answered to test her patience.

"Then you can sit there and use it the rest of your life," she countered with words that stung like a slap in the face.

Whenever she had something bothering her, she spoke her mind and didn't hold back. She got things out of her system immediately.

"Well, maybe I *do* want to use it the rest of my life," I countered.

Cramer didn't appreciate my brainless reply. As she passed my wheelchair to leave, she "accidentally" stepped on my toes.

I yelled, "Ouch. Dammit. Did you do that on purpose?"

With an almost imperceptible smile, she answered, "Would I do that to a patient?"

As I rubbed my toes, I told her, "Yeah, to this patient you would."

She didn't always want to have the last word. One of her favorite ways to win an argument was to walk away and leave you to deal with your own conscience. Nothing was more powerful than that. She often said, "A guilty conscience needs no accuser."

I loved the electric wheelchair. It allowed me to go places and do things I couldn't do otherwise. It was fun to push the joystick full forward and zip along at six miles an hour. It made me more independent. I didn't want to give it up.

Then the lightbulb went off inside my head! I was caught up in the "patient's dilemma." I subconsciously wanted to stay in my familiar way of living and not struggle to reach the next level of improvement.

In intensive care, I had been accused of having the patient's dilemma. Some staff believed I had lost motivation and wasn't trying to improve and described me as "passive." Of course, that was a foolish judgment because my condition at that time was miserable. It wasn't a condition I wanted to stay in if I could change it.

But, now I was at a different level. I was breathing on my own, eating real food, and getting around in an electric wheelchair. Was that enough for me? Was I now truly engaged in the patient's dilemma and satisfied to stay in that condition rather than struggle to improve?

I thought about it. I was reasonably comfortable in my present situation. It accommodated my limitations and I could function well enough to do the basic things I needed to do. Frustrations were minimized because I wasn't pressured to do anything beyond my abilities. If I chose to, I could stay in this stage of development and get by indefinitely.

Trying to improve further meant enduring physical pain and frustration. Stretching my frozen joints was painful. Exercising was hard and full of setbacks. It meant enduring the mental stress of slow progress with its inevitable failures. I'd be forced to try to do things outside my "comfort zone." I'd have to struggle and sweat, experience failure, and disturb my present way of life. I'd have to constantly psych myself up. I wasn't even sure further improvements were possible. It would be much easier to settle for what I had. I was in a protective womb.

My choice was between remaining in my reasonably comfortable situation or struggling for unknown improvements and disturbing my daily routine. Yes, I *was* caught up in the patient's dilemma.

I saw patients go both ways. Some kept trying to improve until they tired of the long struggle and finally said, "To hell with it." They simply couldn't muster the inner strength to keep trying after failing repeatedly. They had reached the limits of their mental endurance. Those patients permanently remained at their existing level and their unused muscles atrophied and forever lost their ability to improve. Some nurses didn't seem to realize that patients could burn out too.

However, other patients kept trying in spite of their ongoing frustrations. They had a stronger inner drive to succeed. I believed that patients had innately different thresholds for dealing with the stresses of longterm rehabilitation.

In my case, I didn't know what my limits were. I believed I could still improve, but I didn't know how much. Many times, I was tempted to quit struggling, but something inside kept urging me to keep on keeping on. I sometimes burned out temporarily, but I always regained my motivation after backing off for a while to let my emotional energy recharge itself. I had a support system of nurses, therapists, and friends who kept me motivated. However, my most important motivation was thinking about my former self-image. I remembered the way I was before my paralysis and that image spurred me on.

I hated being thought of as a cripple and seeing expressions of pity on the faces of others. I wanted to be the way I was—or at least be at a level of functioning I could accept. I knew if I didn't exercise and sat or lay around all day watching television, my muscles would atrophy and my joints would become as stiff as a frozen fish. The inactivity might also result in pneumonia or bedsores. Staying in a comfort zone was a health risk.

In order to stay fully motivated, I needed to be rewarded with noticeable improvements. Each bit of progress was a positive reinforcement, but each failure was a negative reinforcer.

Las Vegas slot machines paid off just enough to keep the players feeding coins. If there wasn't enough positive reinforcement, people stopped playing. Exercising wasn't giving me enough payoffs. I often thought of quitting. It took guts to keep trying after experiencing failure after failure.

All these thoughts were mixed together in my mind in a crazy patchwork of conflicting emotions. To be or not to be, that was the question, whether it was nobler of my mind to suffer the pain and suffering of my outrageous misfortune, or exercise my legs and arms, and in so doing, strengthen them.

Cramer had made her point. She was right—as usual. I got the message and reluctantly returned the electric wheelchair to Judy the next day. From then on, whether I liked it or not, I'd have to let Wilson push me around while I kept trying to push myself.

One afternoon, as I was sitting in my wheelchair in the hallway outside my room, I thought I'd try to see if I could push on my wheelchair's wheels and make it move. I placed my hands on the wheels and pushed half-heartedly. The chair didn't move.

Mrs. Cramer saw what I was trying to do and said firmly, "Try again Mr. Sweeta. If yuh nebba fail, it's cause ya ain't tryin to do."

I made another effort to push against the wheels, but my wheelchair still didn't budge.

"How about a little help Mrs. Cramer."

Instead of helping, she scolded me, "Try harder, you quitter."

I wasn't really annoyed by her name-calling, but I responded with pretended anger.

"Slave driver."

"You're just lazy," she countered.

"Tyrant," I shot back at her.

"Yankee." She liked to call me that when I bothered her.

"Foreigner," I gave it back.

"Empty barrel mek de mos nize."

"Oh, so now we're back to Jamaican talk, eh? Well, individuals who reside in vitric edifices should not hurl projectiles."

"Wat dat mean, Yankee?"

"It means, people who live in glass houses shouldn't throw stones."

"Oh yeah, fishaman nebba say im fish stink."

Cramer wanted an answer. She was enjoying the contest.

"Your turn, you roguin Joe."

151

I sighed, "I give up. I'm done."

Sensing victory, she agreed. "Ooo laff las, laff bess."

We both burst out laughing. It was just two good friends letting off a little steam.

Cramer had different laughs for different situations. There was her polite laughter for most occasions, a girlish giggle when she felt a little embarrassed, and a guttural laugh from deep within when she was really amused—like now.

She walked away and left me sitting in the hallway. I sat there for a while doing nothing. I wanted to go back into my room and watch television, but there was no one around to help me. My TV was on and I could hear one of my favorite shows was on. I put my hands on the wheels and pushed down hard. Nothing happened. I really wanted to watch the show, so I pushed again with every ounce of strength I had. I detected a very slight movement of the chair. I pushed real hard again. The chair moved an inch.

I told myself, "All right John, you moved one inch, you can move another inch." I did. It took all the strength I could muster, but I moved inch by hard-fought inch. After ten hard minutes, I was back in my room. I was completely exhausted but very proud of myself. I eagerly looked forward to Cramer's praise for my accomplishment.

A minute later, she came into my room. She had been watching my struggle without my knowing.

"Well, I'm glad to see you finally got in your room by yourself, but you're as slow as a parson quine to hell. You'll do better next time."

That was Cramer. She acknowledged my accomplishment in her way—and I understood. Her slight smile and indirect words of praise were all I needed. I had my reward and she had hers.

Within a few weeks, I was able to wheel myself around.

Each small bit of progress led to the next. I had been trying to touch my face for a long time, but I couldn't bend my elbow enough to enable me to scratch my face when it itched. When dust or lint got in my nose, I had to stoically bear it. One day while raising my hand to try to touch my face, my thumb contacted my mouth and nose. It was the first time in over a year I had touched my own face. It felt great. I kept touching my face with my thumb as I said, "Hello nose, hello mouth."

I repeated the words to myself over and over, enjoying my new accomplishment. I could finally scratch my nose and face and not have to endure the maddening itching. It was wonderful. Maybe soon I'd be able to feed myself.

However, Cramer wasn't satisfied with the range of motion in my shoulders. They were still mostly frozen with contractures and had minimal rotation. She realized the therapists had limited time to work on my joints, so she went to Doug, the physical therapy supervisor, and asked him for instructions on how to work on my shoulder contractures.

Each morning after bedbaths, she gave me the range of motion exercises Doug had taught her. It took extra time and effort, but she did it willingly. Cramer was going way beyond the call of duty.

One morning while she was manipulating my arm and shoulder, there was a horribly loud cracking sound. She stopped immediately. We were both shook up. We thought she had snapped a bone.

She gingerly rotated my shoulder to assess the damage. Neither of us knew what to expect. I felt no pain as she moved my arm. The arm rotated more than it had previously.

It turned out that the noise was the sound of the ligaments and tendons breaking free. No harm had been done and my arm had almost full rotation. We looked at each other and sighed with relief.

Inspired by her success, Cramer repeated the process on the other shoulder. It also snapped, crackled, and popped. Success again. In following days of manipulation, my shoulder rotation improved to its full range. My shoulders had been unfrozen by a nurse who dared to take on a difficult and intimidating task because that was the only way she knew how to nurse—totally.

The mobility of my shoulders had another positive effect. I could now feed myself by wedging a spoon between my fingers and raising it to my mouth. That was a major accomplishment.

One morning after my PT session with Rick, I struck up a conversation with Doug, the physical therapy supervisor. Doug was a soft-spoken black man of about fifty with the muscular body of an athlete. He sat down in a chair next to me and began massaging my hands while we talked. He had exceptionally strong hands and I wished he were my occupational therapist so he could work the contractures out of my joints. The job required someone with his strength.

As he massaged my hands, I thought I'd get Doug's opinion on how much exercise I should be doing. I didn't mention it to him, but the doctor in charge of the PT department had told me that with Guillain Barré, it was detrimental to overtire myself and had advised me to take it slow and easy. I remembered how my exhaustion just before the onset of my paralysis had played a part in breaking down my body's defense system. But, I still had doubts about the dividing line between too much and not enough exercise.

Doug's answer was, "John, do as much exercise as you can. The longer your muscles are unused, the greater the risk they will atrophy. So, work hard with Rick and keep your muscles stimulated."

His advice made sense. I decided that's what I would do. Even though my rehabilitation was progressing, it was maddeningly slow. Serious doubts of whether I would fully recover lingered in the back of my mind. Would I ever walk normally again? Use my hands? Speak clearly? Will I plateau at some point and remain permanently handicapped? If that happened, what would I do? Could I mentally accept it and make the most of my life, or would I sink into a life of despair? The possibilities were frightening.

I couldn't hold back from telling Doug about my anxieties.

"Doug, I know I've improved some, but I've still got such a long way to go that I get depressed. I hate being so dependent on others for every little thing. I try hard not to think of myself as handicapped because the word makes me think of myself as a crippled, helpless person."

Doug kept massaging my fingers, bending the joints as far as they would go, trying to increase the range of motion. He didn't say anything for a few minutes, but I could tell he was carefully thinking about how to answer me.

Finally, he broke the silence. "John, what if I told you that everyone is handicapped in one way or another?"

"C'mon, Doug. What are you talking about? You aren't handicapped."

"Sure I am. I was a very good gymnast in college and I had thoughts of making the Olympic team, but I wasn't quite good enough. No matter how hard I trained, I couldn't do what the better gymnasts could do. I was handicapped by my physical limitations."

I replied, "That's not what I call handicapped, Doug. You could still do the everyday things normal people do."

He continued, "Okay, let's analyze what being judged handicapped really means. People not only have a wide range of physical abilities, but they also differ in how well they do them. For example, if you're a so-called "normal" person but your vision isn't 20-20 even with glasses, are you handicapped? Can't walk long distances? Poor memory? Do any of those things mean you're handicapped? Yes, those things are handicaps, but you still aren't considered a handicapped person. "

I reponded. "That's true, Doug."

"John, A person is usually described as handicapped if his problem is *visible*, like using a wheelchair, having a missing limb, or simply being old and feeble. I know it's unfair, but a lot of our definition of handicapped is based on appearance rather than functional ability. People who are not visibly handicapped aren't usually judged by others as handicapped—even if they have a serious unseen physical disability, like heart trouble or emphysema. However, it doesn't seem to matter whether a person is completely functional or not, he is still judged handicapped if he *looks* handicapped. Right or wrong, that's simply the way people think. The answer is to realize we're all different in our abilities, so focus on all the things you *can* do, and not be concerned with a label."

That was his message to me. He finished massaging my hands and placed them back in my lap. It was a signal he was also finished with his advice.

"Thanks, Doug. I understand what you're saying." We smiled at each other as I wheeled myself out of the gym.

On the way back to my room, I recalled what Doug had said. Everyone had some type of physical limitation. A visible physical impairment was the criterion people used to define a handicapped person, even if the person could fully function without needing anyone else's help. Therefore, if I left the hospital on a walker, I would be seen by others as handicapped—regardless of whether I could dress and feed myself, drive a car, work at a job, and fully function in the outside world.

I understood that some people would treat my disability with compassion, but others might see my handicap as unpleasant because it was uncomfortable to be around someone who didn't do things like everyone else. Some people might wish I'd just go away. Judgments of handicapped people could be unfair—even cruel at times—but that's the way it was and I'd have to learn to deal with it. I had no control of how people reacted to my disability, but I could control how I responded to them. I decided that when I left the hospital, if I hadn't fully recovered, the quality of my life wouldn't be any less than if I had no disability.

Life was all about attitude, how I chose to think about things. I had the choice of whether to be grateful for all the things I could do or dwell on things I couldn't that didn't really matter. I'd try to remember my darkest hours and how far I had come.

Meanwhile, I continued making progress walking between the parallel bars until I could walk nine lengths without Rick's help.

Rick suggested I try using a walker. I agreed and he brought one over to me. It had wheels on the front, so all I had to do was push it by shuffling my feet forward. I managed to move forward a few steps without any problem.

The walker was sent to my ward for me to use whenever I wanted. Soon I was able to stand up and get in the walker by myself. The independence of exercising on my own felt great. I didn't have to depend totally on Rick anymore.

However, using the walker required courage. It was scary to get on the walker and leave the security of my wheelchair. No one was standing by to grab me if I fell. I didn't know what I would do if I tired and couldn't get back to my chair. It took confidence to walk away from the wheelchair and beyond the sight of nurses. I was taking a chance and had to control my fear.

In order to gain the confidence I needed, I silently repeated positive affirmations to myself every afternoon while sunbathing on the patio outside my room. I repeated the encouraging words over and over in my mind. They must have had an effect because each day I dared to walk farther and farther away from my wheelchair's security.

Each afternoon, after I said my positive affirmations, I relaxed in my wheelchair on the patio and closed my eyes with my face to the sun. It felt warm and soothing. The rays seemed to penetrate my skin and go deep inside my bones. A slight smile was usually on my lips as I dozed off.

One afternoon, I was suddenly wakened from my reverie when I felt something on my nose. Calmly, I half-opened one eye to see what the object was. It was a bee !

"Whoa," I blurted out. My natural fear of being stung made me instinctively brush him off. He took to flight as I sat up straight. I waited to see what he would do about my hostile action.

He circled around me a few times, then landed gently on my arm. He didn't seem irritated or angry so I let him stay till I decided what to do with him. I didn't want to kill him; I just wanted to get rid of him and resume my peaceful sunbathing.

I raised my arm and blew air at him. He didn't move. I blew harder and harder until his wings fluttered from my wind. However, he wasn't disturbed. He seemed to be content on my arm, enjoying the sunshine just as I had been.

I didn't want to leave him on my arm because I couldn't be sure he wouldn't sting me, so I carefully bent over and, with my opposite hand, managed to pick up a small leaf lying on the cement. Nudging him with the leaf didn't seem to bother him and make him fly off. He simply walked onto it as I slid it under him. Raising the leaf to eye level, I studied him for a few minutes. He was a rather small and unscary bee. A nice, likeable bee. Not buzzing and flitting around, just lazily sitting on the leaf, minding his own business.

I accidentally dropped the leaf with the bee still on it. I looked down but couldn't see him on the cement. I turned my head to check around my wheelchair. No luck. Where was he? I rolled my wheelchair around to check further. As the left wheel came around, I saw my little friend, half crushed and stuck on the wheel. He must have been under my wheel and when I turned the chair, it rolled over him. Half crushed, he fell off the wheel and lay limp on the cement, not moving.

A sadness came over me. Witnessing so much suffering in the hospital made me hate the death of any living thing, including my little bee. He had been a nice bee, just trying to enjoy a Spring afternoon. I wished he could wake up and fly away free like he was meant to do. One minute he was content in the warm sunshine just like me, and the next minute he was lifeless. Death could be so senseless....

Edwin's death was senseless too.

I first met Edwin in the gym. He was sitting in a wheelchair next to mine, waiting for a volunteer to push him back to his room. We introduced ourselves and from his manner of speaking, I could tell Ed was an educated man, probably around forty-five years old. During our conversation, Ed told me he had Lou Gehrig's disease and it was causing the progressive loss of his muscular functioning. I knew ALS was fatal and there was no cure, but I tried not to show my concern.

In turn, I told Ed that I was also fighting paralysis from Guillain Barré. In a true gesture of kindness, he said he knew others who had my illness and were now fully recovered. It was incredibly generous of him to try to comfort me when his own condition was so much worse.

He returned to his ward, but I saw Ed each day after that because our PT appointments were at the same time. During our many conversations, we exchanged personal information about our prior lives and we became close friends.

He told me he had been a highschool English teacher and expressed how much he missed teaching and being around young people. With pride, he related how he used to enjoy dressing up in suits and sportscoats for classes. I identified with what he was saying and told him I used to take pride in dressing well myself. We laughed as we looked at each other wearing crumpled hospital pajamas, a far cry from the persons we had been.

In spite of his severe illness, Ed was certain he would fully recover. His optimism was admirable, though unrealistic. He kept a smile on his face despite the pain he was suffering. He simply would not allow himself to dwell on negative thoughts and maintained an unwavering belief that his positive attitude would somehow overcome his debilitating disease.

I would have liked to believe in that power too, but after many months in the hospital, I had watched some of the most positive thinkers I had ever known succumb to their illnesses. Obviously, if all it took was a positive mental attitude to stay healthy or cure a disease, we'd all live forever—but we don't. When Mother Nature calls, we go.

However, I did not think that that was a reason to just give up and wallow in self-pity.Thinking positively gave me the spirit to fight and do things that contributed to my health, like exercising, eating properly, and not dwelling on dark thoughts.

One day, Ed mentioned he had read an article about the future possibility of brain and spinal column transplants. He desperately wanted to believe that some miracle operation might offer a way out of his desperate situation. At first, I thought he was joking about such an implausible operation, but I realized he was serious. Even an intelligent man like Ed would grasp at any ray of hope, however unlikely. Hope did "spring eternal in the human breast."

As his condition worsened through the following weeks, I saw that Ed needed something to bolster his spirits, so one day I suggested he could teach English to some of the foreign-born patients and staff. He could conduct bedside classes. The idea appealed to him and his eyes began to sparkle. He wanted to teach in spite of his pain, muscle weakness, and shortness of breath.

The next day, I carefully handprinted some fliers and posted them on bulletin boards around the hospital. In a few days, Ed had a number of patients stopping by his bed for tutoring. He was a teacher once again and loving every minute of it!

Ed taught English to patients for a few months, until his voice became too weak and his general health deteriorated. He wasn't able to exercise in the gym anymore, so I visited him in his room. He managed to tell me in whispered tones that his only remaining pleasure was in his sleep when he dreamed he was healthy and teaching at his old highschool.

He quoted from his teachings, "Into the land of dreams I long to go."

I wanted to tell Edwin that I used to escape into dreams too--but his escape was different. Mine were a temporary way of gaining relief—his dreams were the only relief he would ever have.

His dreams were nature's way of symbolically unloading all the fears his mind had repressed. It was a purification process. They also allowed Ed to have his wishes fulfilled in the land of the subconscious.

At this point, Ed realized there would be no miracle cure for him. He was resigned to his fate. He had accepted his mortality.

I visited Ed every evening and watched him slowly succumbing to his illness. Finally, one evening Ed left this world for a better place. ALS stole his life, but not his dignity.

When Ed died, I silently recited the eulogy I had written for my father when he died:

"As your still body slips beneath the waves, I hear a clarion voice calling your name above the mournful grieving,

"It speaks of your good deeds both great and small, your misfortunes endured with grace, and a worthwhile life lived with no regrets,

"Though your earthly self slowly descends through the dark waters and gently settles in its final resting place,

"Your ethereal self ascends to unimaginable heights and finds eternal peace. So be it. Farewell...."

Chapter 21

Cautious Optimism

"We are about as happy as we make up our minds to be."
Abraham Lincoln

The weeks passed and it was Christmastime again—my second in the hospital. The ward was decorated simply with a small tree and a few banners, but there was a special feeling in the air.

Last Christmas had been a lonely time, but this year was filled with people. Hugh brought my son Chris and they spent Christmas Eve with me. A few people from Western Industries paid a friendly visit on Christmas day. Virginia and Bill sat with me for an hour. Carolers from nearby highschools strolled the halls and the Salvation Army band played and distributed gifts. The VFW gave gift certificates for the canteen, and I received a phone call from Dave Williams, my best friend in Detroit. He didn't know if I'd be penniless when I left the hospital so he offered financial help if I needed it.

I exchanged holiday greetings with dozens of people and chatted with Cramer, Agard, Redden, Hunt, Maryann, and the other nurses. Charlie played Christmas songs and we all sang along. It was a day filled with music, joy, and affection.

This Christmas was all about people sharing feelings and expressing a special warmth they didn't express during the rest of the year. Being in the hospital made it even more meaningful. The holiday spirit allowed everyone to drop their façades and step out of their roles as patient and staff and connect with each other at the deepest human level.

That evening, after the last "Merry Christmas" had been said, I felt exhilarated but tired. The day had been a peak experience, one of those rare and special times that I wished would never end. But, as someone once said, "Don't be sad a wonderful time is over, be happy that you had it." It had been a great Christmas. However, I was exhausted and once in bed, I fell asleep as soon as I closed my eyes.

The week between Christmas and New Years rolled by, and before I knew it, it was the start of a brand new year. I couldn't help wondering if this was my year to leave the hospital. The thought was exciting and scary at the same time.

I saw improvements in my physical condition, but I was hesitant to read too much optimism into them. I had progressed from walking short distances in the walker to walking so far I didn't know what my limit was. I could turn myself in bed, exercise by myself in the gym, and do many other things, but I didn't allow myself to become overly hopeful.

I asked myself why I was reluctant to feel more optimistic. Was I in a state of denial or was I afraid I might be setting myself up for a huge disappointment if my progress suddenly stopped? I still had a long way to go before I could function outside the hospital.

I also didn't want to fully accept the slow improvement that disagreed with my original hope that my paralysis would one day reverse itself in one massive turnaround and not in these small steps. The belief in a quick turnaround still lingered in the back of my mind, regardless of the reality of what was actually happening. My thoughts remained cautious.

Whenever I felt depressed about my slow progress, Cramer was there to support me. She often quoted, "The race is not to the swiftest, but to him who persists to the end."

She understood my periods of depression and realized I couldn't always be cheerful and upbeat---that everyone has days when they feel down. So, whenever I became frustrated, she allowed me to vent my anger, knowing I couldn't mentally pump myself up day after day without having some bad days in between.

Cramer said, "No one is cheerful all the time. Who would want to be in that giddy state of mind constantly?"

She was right. I recalled that George Bernard Shaw had said, "No man alive could bear a lifetime of happiness, it would be hell on earth."

My mind seemed to be in a constant battle between positive thoughts of a quick recovery and negative thoughts of a slow recovery. My mood swung back and forth like a pendulum. These two inner opposing forces were what the philosopher Goethe had described as the mind's "two souls within my breast struggling for undivided reign."

So, I got to thinking. "Just what is that inner demon inside my head that makes me so negative and self-destructive? Is that demon a part of the "real me" or is it some outer spiritual force like religion's devil invading my mind? Where does it happen in my brain? *Why* is it in my brain?"

I knew from a biology class I had taken that stimulation of the brain's pleasure-center caused the brain to secrete serotonin or dopamine, the "feel-good" chemicals. In the class laboratory, I had implanted an electrode in a rat's hypothalamus and connected it to a lever with a switch. When the rat pressed the lever, it received an electrical stimulation. The rat pressed the lever relentlessly for the pleasant feeling it received.

In contrast, I had read that stimulation of a monkey's amygdalae triggered chemicals that caused uncontrolled rage and aggression—the energy of nature's survival instinct. Removal of the monkey's amygdalae left it tame and docile.

Since both pleasurable feelings and aggression could be turned on by an electrical stimulus to those primitive areas of the brain, it showed that both emotions were natural to the brain's functioning. Similarly in humans, those regions were shown by computer imagery to be activated during those same emotions. Both centers were just a part of a person's natural physiology. Simple enough. No mystery there.

I said to myself, "Okay, it's nice to have the positive, constructive, feel-good glands, but why do the powerful glands that supply necessary survival energy also cause negative, self-destructive thinking?"

As with so many functions in the human body, I knew there needed to be a balance, the Yin and the Yang. Why shouldn't positive thinking be balanced with negative thinking?They were nature's positive and negative polarities, the anode and cathode that make us all bipolar in varying degrees. Wasn't it necessary to have both? Maybe it was good for me to have a negative shaking out process every so often to unload all the frustrations that had accumulated in my mind.

However, both a state of hyper-elation or hyper-negativity could be psychologically harmful. Uninterrupted mania would be exhausting and ultimately lead to a breakdown in the system's balance. Without a negative counter-balance, the mind would constantly be thinking excited, everything-is-wonderful thoughts with no concern for possible harmful consequences--leading to cautionless, reckless, foolish pursuits that were blind to dangers and might even be fatal. Fears and doubts kept the mind grounded in reality and prevented irrational manic behaviors. They served a survival purpose.

On the other hand, too much negativity could be harmful. Self-doubt, anxiety, and fears had to be kept in check in order to maintain a rational, balanced state of mind. Excessive negative, aggressive energy produced by the limbic system had to be expressed somehow to relieve the pressure. If not released outwardly, it would turn inwardly against the self in the form of pessimism, self-hatred, and depression. Strangely, even an attack against the self could sometimes give a masochistic feeling of pleasure because of the release of the pent up energy—an example of the mind's complex pleasure-pain balance.

I knew that was where the rational part of my brain, the prefrontal cortex, came into play. Instead of seeing negativity as a destructive "demon" inside of me, something I despised and didn't accept nor want, I believed I should see it as an essential part of my brain's normal functioning. I believed I should make friends with my "other" self, talk to it, get to understand it, accept it as much a part of "me" as my positive thinking, and see it as part of nature's grand scheme of things.

But, I knew excessive aggressive energy had to be controlled by diverting it outwardly away from the self—not by using the energy against others through social aggression or violence, but by expressing it in acceptable ways. It could be displaced by venting it through vigorous physical activities such as exercise, competitive sports either personally or vicariously, or engaging in any strenuous physical labors or chores. It's powerful energy could also be released through sublimation, providing the aggressive drive, the fighting spirit, and the determined will to accomplish personal goals. The possible outlets were endless.

Problems only arose when the rational mind did not have the control to keep the conflicting energies in balance. Freud's id-ego-superego interaction explained it more fully.

For my rehabilitaton, I needed the positive energy to keep me motivated and I needed the negative energy to fuel my muscles for aggressive exercising and improving my strength. A nice working relationship. As long as I maintained a regular daily routine of exercise and other outlets, I could stop over-analyzing because the balance would take care of itself.

Cramer was right about not having to always think only cheerful, positive thoughts. I didn't want to pretend everything was okay when it wasn't. Otherwise, I wouldn't face my problems and try to correct them.

Also, the pressure to always be upbeat could make me feel guilty whenever my positive attitude didn't result in the progress I expected, Was it my fault for not thinking positively enough? I didn't need that burden of guilt. I didn't want to chastise myself every time my progress didn't meet expectations based on the false belief that my positive attitude would automatically lead to improvements and negativism automatically led to setbacks.

I could see where obsessive, positive thinking was temporarily motivating, but it didn't apply to my situation. The glowing feeling of inner power might shine brightly for a short while, but would soon burn itself out like a flashbulb. Mental highs could quickly evaporate and turn into mental lows.

For me to cope with my rehabilitation, I had to focus on the long term—not pump myself up like a kid at a highschool pep rally. I needed to blend a controlled, longterm, balanced state of mind with realistic expectations. That was the secret.

That delicate balance meant constant self-awareness. It meant avoiding extreme elation using self-control developed through daily positive affirmations, and by avoiding extreme negativity through displacement and sublimation when aggressive energy became self-defeating. I didn't need all the psycho-babble of overly complicated "therapies." My rational brain was the moderator, even though it understandably could not always be wise enough to keep the peaceful balance. There would always be times of too much emotion one way or the other.

I knew the future would be a challenge and I'd have Goethe's battle of two inner souls to deal with for the rest of my life. I would always have mood swings when the inner juices were flowing, but I'd do my best to keep my emotions balanced. So be it.

A patient in the room next to me, was a perfect example of a someone who constantly had a cheerful attitude—unfortunately.

Frank was a handsome, middle-aged fellow. He was the nicest guy you'd ever want to meet, always friendly, always smiling, always showing an upbeat, pleasant self. He had a minor case of Guillain Barré which partially paralyzed his hands. I figured he'd stay in the hospital for a few weeks of physical therapy instruction, then be discharged. Lucky guy.

All the nurses loved Frank. Who wouldn't? I did too, at first. He was extremely polite and complimentary to everyone. But, after a few days, his cheerfulness began to wear on me. Everything he said was repetitious and syrupy. In a short time, his cloying niceness became irritating.

I began to wonder if Frank had a real personality. There was no color to him, no character. He was always the same, no lows, no depression, no anger, no bitterness—no anything but a cheerful, pleasant attitude. He was probably the ideal patient that nurses always hoped for.

How could I interact with a guy like Frank who was always smiling and could only hold superficial conversations? There was no depth to him. Talking with him was unnatural.

In the following weeks, Frank's partially paralyzed hands improved and he didn't require further hospitalization so he was scheduled for discharge. Before he left, he came to my room to say goodbye. However, in saying farewell, Frank stopped smiling for a moment and his expression became serious for the first time. He admitted to me that he often felt depressed but hid it from everyone because he thought a "good" patient wasn't supposed to complain or show his true feelings. He had kept his emotions in check and put on a smiley face.

At that moment, I connected with Frank. He was a real person after all. I felt his psychological pain and I was sad he hadn't allowed himself to show his humanity.

The nurses had never been aware of his secret feelings. After he left, I overheard nurses say, "I miss Frank, he was no trouble at all," and "I wish all the patients were like Frank."

I wondered if that were true. Did nurses really want robots for patients? If all patients acted like Frank, nurses would never develop professionally or personally. If nurses were never challenged, they would stay at the same level of nursing as when they started. Without the ups and downs of human interaction, they would never improve their skills. Dealing with a patient's full range of emotions was difficult, but it was the source of a nurse's greatest rewards and personal growth— whether she realized it or not. It was just as important as dealing with a patient's physical problems—maybe more so.

Frank left and the nurses never had a chance to see his true inner self and help him deal with his fears and anxieties. It was a sad ending that wouldn't have happened if Frank had allowed himself to just be human.

On the other hand, there was Mr. Johnson. He gave the nurses a lot of practice in how to deal with a difficult patient. His aggressive energy ran wild. He was the exact opposite of Frank. Mr. Johnson was obnoxious. All day long, he yelled, "Nurse," "Nurse." When they came, he cussed them out with crude obscenities. Cramer assigned him to only the most experienced nurses. I couldn't understand how they were able to take so much verbal abuse without responding harshly. The tolerance they showed for such an obnoxious patient was commendable.

One nurse said the uneducated patients used more profanity. I saw her point because two of the more obnoxious patients had been homeless men living on the streets. They not only cursed the nurses, but they expected royal treatment, demanding better food, a private bath, and special drapes on the windows. I couldn't believe their gall.

My friend, Murphy, had also cussed out nurses and patients alike until the day a patient he bad-mouthed took a glass of water and threw it in his face. Drenched in cold water, Murphy shut up. He never swore at that patient again and started to tone down his language with everyone.

I wondered whether that wasn't a useful behavior modification technique. If nurses flicked just a little cold water into a patient's face when he used strong profanity, possibly he would learn to associate cursing with a cold water shock and be conditioned away from cursing. But, even if it worked, I knew hospitals would never allow it.

A patient in the gym often used foul language with a therapist. One day, the patient became violent and slapped the therapist. I suggested to the therapist that he might try a little aversive therapy by loudly yelling "NO" to startle him whenever he got out of control. He said he understood why the patient was acting out and he would restrain the patient's arms if he ever felt it was necessary. And that was that.

It still bothered me to see nurses and therapists used as targets for patients' uncontrolled anger. A few times I interceded and told the patients to settle down and shut up. I could say things to them that the staff couldn't.

When I asked nurses how they put up with so much verbal abuse, their usual replies were, "The patient is sick and doesn't know what he's saying," or "I don't let it bother me."

I asked Cramer how she dealt with patients swearing at her. She had her own style of dealing with them—as usual.

She said, "I completely excuse a patient who is delusional or in pain. I understand some are cursing out of frustration and anger. Nevertheless, when a patient is not delusional and is too far out-of-line, I look him straight in the eye and tell him, 'You will not use that kind of language on this ward, do you understand!?' I do not stop eyeballing him until he realizes I'm not fooling and he backs down. Bullies always do."

I had received that unblinking stare a few times and I knew that eyeball-to-eyeball stare of hers could freeze your lips shut.

Cramer continued, "Once they acknowledge that I will not tolerate abusive language, they apologize and stop cursing. Nevertheless, all patients receive the same good care, no matter how they behave."

She topped it off with penetrating Jamaican wisdom, "Cuss-cuss no bore hole inna man skin. Dey know yuh canna sid pon horse back an curse horse."

What could I say to such uncomplicated reasoning.

I wondered why nurses didn't get the same respect they got in the past. What had changed? Was it because our society was now less civilized? Was it somehow related to the casual dress most nurses wore these days that changed patients' perceptions of them?

Nurses' dress codes had changed drastically in many hospitals, especially the absence of the traditional caps. I had read studies which confirmed the power of uniforms worn by policemen, the military, airline pilots, and others who needed the image of authority. If uniforms had no effect on others' responses to them, no one would wear them. A nurse's uniform established her identity and the conduct expected from patients, doctors, and visitors. Uniforms had served a purpose for centuries.

Uniforms also had an effect on the wearer. They made the wearer identify more with the role and behave accordingly.

The VA Hospital didn't have a firm dress code for ward nurses. As long as it was white, they were allowed to wear any type of clothing they wanted. Some chose to wear dresses, some wore skirts and blouses, others shirts and slacks. It was a mishmash of styles. None wore white stockings and only one nurse in the whole hospital wore a cap. They all looked neat and clean, but without the traditional uniform and cap, they lacked the time-honored look of a nurse. The distinctive cap was like a tiara that distinguished her from people who worked in drugstores, bakeries, and other occupations with white uniforms. Like a nun's headdress, it gave a halo effect that gained respect. Without it, the magic was gone.

The one nurse in the VA hospital who wore a cap, had a wonderful look that the others didn't. I couldn't help smiling my approval every time I saw her. There was no doubt about who she was. She was a nurse.

Whenever I asked nurses why they didn't wear caps, I was told, "They're a nuisance," or "I feel freer," or "That went out with Florence Nightingale." Most were irritated with me for even asking such a "dumb" question. After all, this was a different time.

When Cramer and I discussed the issue, she eye-balled me and said, "Mister, I don't need a cap to get respect."

I told her, "Okay, if the cap isn't important, why wear a uniform at all? Why don't nurses wear sweatshirts, bluejeans, and tennis shoes?"

Cramer didn't respond, so I kept trying to make my point, "I've seen nurses in other hospitals who wear flowered blouses, patterned slacks, and all kinds of casual clothing. It's becoming harder and harder to tell who is a nurse and who isn't. You told me yourself that one of your patients keeps calling the nurses 'waitresses.' I think nurses should go back to the same look that worked so well for over a hundred years. Maybe it's time for nurses' uniforms to get a make-over like the uniforms of nuns and military women have done."

Cramer rolled her eyes, paused for a while, then said, "That's a dumb idea." She started to eye-ball me and I knew I had not made my point. It was time for me to shut up.

I concluded, "Okay, okay, if nothing else, a cap helps hide a bad hair day."

As she turned to leave, I quietly muttered to myself, "I still think I'm right."

She stopped and whirled around, "What did you say?"

I said, "It's all right."

My belief that nurses' uniforms made a big difference in how patients perceived and reacted to them was confirmed a few days later.

Cramer always worked the morning shift and gave me my bedbath. She knew my body as well as I did. Late one evening in her off-duty hours, Cramer came to the ward to finish some paperwork. She had on regular clothing: a knee-length skirt that showed her shapely legs, a sheer silk blouse, and sandals. She had on bright lipstick and more makeup than when she was on duty. I didn't even recognize her at first. All of a sudden, she wasn't a nurse—Cramer was a woman! Without her white nurse's dress, she was a whole different person.

At the time, Mrs. Agard was changing my pajamas because I had spilled food on them. I didn't want Cramer to see me naked. That very morning, Cramer had washed me, toileted me, and dressed me—but now I was embarrassed for her to see me naked. I was glad Agard kept me covered. Instead of relating to Cramer as patient to nurse, it was man to woman. Her clothing totally changed my perception of her. I'm sure she didn't see me differently because I was still in the role of a patient, but I certainly saw her differently.

I knew tomorrow morning Cramer would be in her nurse's outfit again and my attitude would revert back. As I thought about it, the whole experience was ridiculously silly, but that's the way her lack of a uniform affected me.

Sure enough, the next morning, Cramer was in her white nursing dress and our relationship was back to normal.

While Cramer was giving me my bedbath, I asked her if the decubitus had opened up again. The decubitus on my buttock had healed months ago, but sometimes it felt like it had reopened. It hadn't of course, but the scar tissue felt differently than the surrounding skin.

She jabbed her finger hard on the scar.

"Ouch, why did you do that?" I demanded.

She responded, "Did I show you it's okay?"

I realized that I had insulted her nursing care by asking a question that implied she might have been negligent. She made it clear I'd better not ask that question again. I didn't.

After breakfast, Cramer weighed me. I saw my weight was up to 155 pounds. Good food and exercise were doing their jobs.

A little later, Dr. Bruce dropped by to see how my speech was coming along. He could hear I still had a slight slurring caused by the remaining paralysis in my tongue. He invited me to attend speech therapy to see if he couldn't help correct the slurring. During five sessions, he was able to lessen the slurring and we made an instructional video to present to future students in the speech department. I was a video star.

Meanwhile, I was still having questions regarding my physical therapy. How much exercise was beneficial and how much was harmful? The problem was further complicated when one of the rehab doctors was on the ward and gave me advice.

I was sitting in my wheelchair in the hallway outside my room when Dr. Glover passed by and recognized me.

He said, "Hello," but didn't remember my name.

"Hello, Dr. Glover," I answered, showing I remembered his.

"How are you?" Everyone always asked me that. It must be written in their manuals as an opening line with patients.

"Fine, thanks," I replied for the umpteenth time. Did they really want to know? What if I went ahead and gave them a long list of my problems? I wished people would just say hello without asking me how I was.

"Can you move your hands?"

I thought to myself, "Oh no, not that again"

He made a fist with his hand and asked me to do the same.

I thought, "Here we go again."

Everyone seemed to focus on my hands. They always asked me to try and make a fist—which I couldn't. Their requests only served to embarrass me.

I showed him my limited hand movement and we started to discuss exercising. Since he was a rehab doctor, I decided to get his opinion on how much exercise I should be doing.

His answer was, "Do not exercise at all. With Guillain Barré, fatiguing yourself can be harmful. The nerve cells are trying to regenerate and there's no use risking damage until they've had a chance to grow back. Wait until the paralysis has gone and then begin exercising."

Cramer was standing nearby and heard our conversation. When Dr. Glover left, Cramer and I discussed his questionable advice. We couldn't believe our ears. How could I keep my muscles from atrophying further if I didn't use them? Didn't exercise increase blood circulation and help nerve tissue grow?

Not only was this new advice illogical, but it was contrary to the advice I got from the chief rehab doctor who told me to exercise in moderation and the advice I received recently from PT supervisor Doug, a man I greatly respected, who advised me to exercise as much as possible.

What should I do when three "experts" in the field all gave differing advice?

Once again, I had to make my own decision and manage my recovery according to my own gut feelings. It seemed I was forced by necessity to make critical decisions throughout my long hospital stay. Sometimes, my decisions went against medical advice, as when I refused excessive X-rays, blood drawings, antibiotics, and steroids. Sometimes, my decisions were wrong, as when I refused to be turned and caused a decubitus, and later when I fought against removing the trach tube from my throat. But, all in all, my batting average was good.

Now I had to decide on an exercise plan. A good decision required that I first state the problem succinctly. If I couldn't do that, I didn't really understand the problem. Next, I had to list all my alternatives without omitting anything, good or bad. Thirdly, I had to sort through the choices and select the most sensible. Lastly, once I began an exercise plan, I'd have to monitor my results and make necessary changes.

I had already stated the problem by asking, "How much exercise is beneficial?" My alternatives were the three pieces of advice I had received. Now came my choice of which to follow.

My common sense told me, if I didn't exercise at all, further muscle atrophication was inevitable. Even if my nerves later regenerated, there wouldn't be enough working muscles left to do anything useful.

However, if I exercised only moderately, I might be exercising too little and prolonging my recovery.

If I exercised too much, there was the possibility of burning up muscle tissue faster than my body could replenish it. I knew that fatigue was a contributing cause of my paralysis in the beginning because I had physically exhausted myself during the time toxins were invading my body.

Which path should I take? The answer was clear to me. I'd be pragmatic and exercise as much as I felt was beneficial.

Lastly, I'd pay strict attention to my body and watch for signs of tiredness, stiffness, pain, and rate of improvement. If my body told me to ease up a little, I would. Otherwise, I'd continue on a dynamic program of exercise. Except for Guillain Barré, I knew the human body seldom sneaked up without giving a warning of some kind. Therefore, if I paid attention to the signals from my internal monitors, my body would tell me all I needed to know. My direction was set.

In the gym, I was doing well on the walker so Rick brought over a quad-cane for me to try out. He wanted to see if I could transition from the walker to a cane. I was able to use it for about twenty steps before my whole body tired. The trial wasn't successful, but we decided to keep trying.

In the afternoons, I continued with my occupational therapy. While waiting for Judy one day, I had a conversation with another patient. He mentioned he had been in an auto accident and had sustained many injuries, including a broken jaw.

His jaws had previously been wired shut and he had to eat liquid nourishment through a straw. During that time, he said he craved a chilidog above all other food and as soon as he was able to eat, he had had his wife bring him two chilidogs with all the trimmings. Once again, I was amazed by the obsession people had for a chilidog when they hadn't eaten solid food for a while.

As we talked, Judy came over to our table and began massaging my hands. While she worked on my fingers, she taught me something important. I had been waiting for my hands to fully function so I could write letters and keep notes on my progress.

Judy told me,"You can start writing now if you want to."

I questioned, "How? I can't use my right hand well enough."

"You don't write with your hand, John. Your hand merely holds the pen. You write by moving your shoulder. Let's try it and I'll show you what I mean."

She placed a piece of paper in front of me, wedged a pen between my fingers, and told me to try writing by moving my shoulder and arm.

Sure enough, it worked. By moving my shoulder, I could maneuver the pen to write. At first, my handwriting was scribbled, but it smoothed out and became very legible. It was an epiphany. Now I could write to friends and make personal notes. With my newly acquired skill, I began making extensive notes and kept a diary of everything that happened around me. My voluminous notes and the tape recordings I made gave me a complete record of my daily life.

The next day in OT, I had another enlightening experience.

A patient named Mr. Dorsey was sitting in a wheelchair next to mine. We were both waiting for our therapists to finish with their patients. He was a friendly, outgoing fellow and we began discussing our therapy sessions. During our conversation, Mr. Dorsey explained he had multiple sclerosis that was progressively destroying his muscles. He explained he was now a partial quadriplegic and in constant pain. In spite of his dreadful condition, he smiled and seemed at ease. He had a cheerfulness that surprised me, considering his problems.

At one point in the conversation, he mentioned he wrote poetry. I told him I loved poetry and wrote a little poetry myself. When I asked him to recite something he had written, he dug into his wheelchair bag and handed me a piece of folded paper. I opened it up and there was a handwritten poem on it entitled "Thank You Lord."

I thank thee for the sunrise
I thank thee for the rain
I thank thee for the wheat
And for the wholesome grain

I thank thee for the weather
With the wind, hail and sleet
I thank thee for our home
And for the food we eat

I thank thee for thyself
For the joy of what thou art
I thank thee for life itself
I thank thee with all my heart

I was overwhelmed with emotion. Here was a man with a degenerative disease that was painful and deadly. It seemed he had nothing going for him, yet he was in excellent spirits and exuded joy. His religious belief contributed to his positive spirit, but that didn't fully explain why he didn't feel some frustration and bitterness. Wasn't he even a little angry with God or life in general for his miserable condition? Was he an optimistic fool?

Mr. Dorsey wasn't a fool. He was a man who had found meaning in his life. He courageously faced the choice of whether to believe his life was hopeless or else believe it had some value. Instead of bemoaning his misfortune, he chose to focus on the simple, good things he had that gave his life meaning. Once again, I realized that being grateful for what you have is the definition of happiness....

I was inspired by his positive outlook on life. Once again, I was compelled to realize that peace of mind was a matter of attitude. His positive energy was contagious. It rubbed off on me and I went through the rest of the day feeling good about my own life.

Unlike Mr. Dorsey, a patient in the room next to mine, was unable to find an existential reason for living. George Keller was a mobile patient who took daily walks around the hospital. In a way, I envied him for his mobility. During his trips, he usually stopped by my room to say hello.

George had a large bandage on his throat and his voice was raspy, so I suspected he had had a laryngeal operation. Nevertheless, he spoke clearly enough. I didn't know exactly what his illness was, but I thought it might be serious since Cramer had placed him in a private room.

During a visit one day, George decided to tell me his problem, "John, see this bandage on my throat? It covers my cancer surgeries. Unfortunately, the cancer isn't gone and there isn't much more the doctors can do for me. Pretty soon I won't be able to talk or swallow. The pain is starting to get really bad in spite of the medication, and I don't intend to put up with it if it gets any worse."

I was taken aback. I had no idea his condition was that serious.

Keller continued, "I'm thinking of stopping my medications and treatments because they're not helping me."

I felt obligated to say something. "George, wouldn't it be better if you played it out to see what happens? "

He shook his head, "The pain and suffering aren't worth it. I'm a burden to myself and everybody else. It's stupid to hang on just for the sake of prolonging the misery. At some point in time, you have to drop the denial. When you hit a wall where healing fails, it's time to face reality."

I didn't say anything. He was speaking the truth, so there was really nothing to say.

He said with finality, "If there was some hope, even a little, it would be different. But, there isn't. So, I'm just going to let nature take its course."

I wasn't sure what he meant by that. Keller was finished with what he wanted to say, so he turned and left. I felt a great sorrow for him. He was a thoughtful, decent human being who didn't deserve this much suffering. No one did.

During the following weeks, George didn't stop to visit me as he usually did. When he walked past my door, I saw he now had an NG feeding tube in his nose and he was pushing an IV stand with fluid draining into his arm. I assumed he had lost the ability to swallow—and possibly to talk. His facial expression showed the extreme pain he was feeling.

A few days later, when he shuffled past my door, I noticed all his tubes were gone. I asked Cramer what the story was. She told me in plain words, "Mr. Keller has pulled all his tubes out and refuses to have them put back in. He is a rational man so he has the right to refuse treatment if he chooses. His doctors have agreed to follow his wishes."

I saw George pass my door only a few times after that. Each time he looked worse. A week later, Mrs. Cramer informed me Keller had died. I mourned for George, but I was glad his misery was over.

A few patients said it was foolish for Keller to stop treatments and remove the life-sustaining fluids. They felt he should have been brave enough to do everything he could to stay alive. I knew better. George had made his choice not to endure needless pain and suffering. His life had lost its preciousness when the quality had gone and there was no hope for recovery. His act was not the act of a coward. It was an incredibly difficult thing to do and took tremendous courage. It went against the most basic instinct—survival. I was dismayed by self-righteous people who pontificated that terminally ill people didn't have the right to choose when their hopeless lives should end. It was George's life to prolong or end—no one else's.

Bill Henderson was another patient who made a decision about his final days. I used to see Bill in the gym and talk with him, but recently he had stopped exercising because of his deteriorating lungs.

In spite of the fact he had only ten percent of his lungs still functioning, he had a lit cigarette in his mouth when he wheeled himself into my room. He looked haggard.

I said, "Bill, what the hell are you doing smoking?"

He shrugged his shoulders and said, "Look, I probably don't have much time left, so what's the difference?"

"Yeah, but you've got an oxygen tank on your chair and you've got those intake tubes in your nose. Don't you know oxygen is flammable?"

"It's okay, I turned it off."

It was hard for me to understand how someone would continue smoking with lungs so wasted. I guessed he simply wanted to enjoy what time he had left in the manner he chose. He seemed content and resigned to his fate.

In the following days, Bill's condition got worse and he was sent to a nursing home. I never saw him after that.

I remembered an experiment I had done in college with a white rat in the laboratory. When I placed the rat in water, it swam. But, if I held it tightly in my hand till it felt helpless and stopped struggling, then put my hand in the water and slowly released my grip, the rat remained limp and would have drowned if I hadn't saved it. It had lost hope and the will to live.

I imagined Keller and Henderson had reached the same point of helplessness and hopelessness. Once they felt unable to do anything to help themselves, they lost their fighting spirit and surrendered.

It was obvious to me that patients made personal choices of whether to fight against their illness, regardless of its severity, or else decided to quit fighting and made peace with their mortality by allowing nature to take its course. It would have been wrong of me to make sanctimonious judgments about the choices desperate men made about their own lives and deaths.

Chapter 22

Psychology or Psycho-Babble?

"I have studied now philosophy and jurisprudence,
medicine and even alas, theology from end to end
and with labor keen, and here, poor fool, with all
my lore, I stand no wiser than before."
Faust, by Johann Wolfgang von Goethe

One morning, a young man in a white coat came into my room and introduced himself as Dr. Strak. He was a psychologist who was completing his licensing practicum at the hospital. He looked like he was in his mid-twenties and was filled with youthful enthusiasm. He asked me if I would be willing to discuss my illness and any problems I might have.

I had nothing to lose, so I agreed to talk with him and see what advice he had to offer. Dr. Strak began by asking me to describe my life before my illness and the events leading up to the paralysis.

Strak listened attentively as I described in detail the life I had led with a good job, a nice home near the beach, and many friends. When I finished, he asked, "Prior to the paralysis, you seemed to be living a very nice life. I'm wondering whether you might have felt a little guilty or uneasy about having such good fortune?"

I replied, "I wasn't feeling guilty at all. I was rather enjoying my life."

Strak interrupted, "Mr. Sueta, sometimes an illness fills a need in a person's life. Your hospitalization removed you from your previous life, so could it be serving a purpose? Was there some stressful situation occurring in your life before your illness?"

It was a logical question. However, why did there have to be a deep, dark subconscious reason for my illness? Why try to make me feel guilty that I had caused my own illness? People already spend too much time on feeling guilty about everything, why add more guilt? I simply had handled toxic chemicals which triggered my immune system into doing what it was supposed to do—but it overreacted.

His psychosomatic illness theory was a stretch, but I was never one to avoid a challenge, so I was willing to explore it for the mental exercise.

"Nothing special happened that I can think of. I'd certainly remember a traumatic situation if there had been one."

Strak wasn't satisfied and asked the same question in a different way. "Mr. Sueta, hospitalization physically removed you from your surroundings and offered you a chance to rest and receive caring attention. Is that something you possibly needed at the time?"

I answered him honestly, "I was living a life with normal stresses and my hospitalization didn't bring me the kind of rest and attention anyone could possibly want. In fact, my hospitalization disrupted a pleasurable life and substituted an incredibly miserable one."

Undaunted, he again rephrased his question, "Yes, but here in the hospital, you get a break from the stresses of the real world. Hasn't that separation been a relief?"

"Dr. Strak, do I look like I'm separated from reality? In the hospital, life is as real as it gets. I face reality every minute of every day. What could be more real than what I'm going through?"

I couldn't help smiling at his persistent attempts to attach a psychological cause to my situation. Because the paralysis had come on quickly and had no established medical basis, Strak wanted to find a psychological causation. He was desperately trying to find the "real" cause for my condition so he could put a label on it and fit it into one of his theories.

Strak had an unquestioning belief in his psychosomatic theory. He wasn't fazed by my arguments to the contrary. I don't think a thunderous voice from God telling him he was on the wrong track would have penetrated his narrow reasoning.

I didn't need the guilt trip of feeling I had caused my own illness. Our first meeting ended in a stalemate.

After Strak left, it was time for my PT appointment. I wheeled myself to the gym. Rick was busy, so I sat and waited. While waiting for Rick, I had a sudden urge to urinate. The urge came on quickly and powerfully. One minute I felt no need to relieve myself and the next minute I had to go so badly I could barely hold it.

I excitedly called Rick over and told him I needed to get to a bathroom fast. After listening to my description of how the urge came on so quickly, he said I was just feeling the "pissing syndrome." He said if I relaxed, the urge would go away. I had never heard of that before. It felt real to me. As much as I needed immediate relief, I thought I'd give it a try. If I let it go, Rick would have to clean it up.

But, he was right. After relaxing for a few minutes, the urge slowly subsided and my need to urinate disappeared, just as Rick had said.

An hour later, after I had finished exercising and was back in my room, I used the bathroom.

Many times after that, whenever I had a very sudden urge to urinate, I relaxed until the urge went away and I waited until a bathroom was handy. I now could tell the difference between a real call of Nature and the "pissing syndrome."

Later that day, Jim from AA staggered into my room. I hadn't seen him for weeks. He was drunk, disheveled, and blubbering like a baby. He looked his usual, pitiful self. Obviously, Jim couldn't stay away from alcohol and it had total control of him. It was depressing to see someone who had once led a productive life fall into the grip of alcoholism. He was stuck on the first rung of the twelve step ladder that lead out of his dark pit.

Jim told me he had been sleeping in the large bushy area on the hospital grounds, but lately he found a porta-potty used by hospital construction workers and he was sleeping in that. He related how other homeless people were sleeping in the hospital closets, therapy rooms, or any unoccupied rooms during the night and using the hospital's bathroom to toilet and wash. They had nowhere else to go.

Jim asked me if I had any spare change. I gave him a few dollars, hoping he would buy something to eat—but I doubted he would use it for food. Sobbing and unable to speak, he staggered out.

I hoped Jim would visit me again. Maybe I could help him in some small way. I didn't know how, but I'd try.

During the week, a series of minor incidents occurred and I couldn't seem to control the negativity. Those petty frustrations had accumulated and the negative energy had turned inward. My gloomy mood got worse when I thought about how my long, hard efforts hadn't resulted in enough improvements to leave the hospital. I worried that my progress would stop before I had recovered to an acceptable level.

My despondent feelings became so strong that I didn't feel like doing anything. It was one of those times I knew would occur when negativity was in control because I somehow hadn't released it either physically or mentally. The balance was out of kilter.

Mrs. Cramer came by for her usual afternoon talk and sensed my bad mood. She asked what was bothering me.

I answered angrily, "I can't keep pumping myself up, Cramer. I've gone to the well too often, it's dry."

She said, "Yes, Mr. Sweeta, ebery day bucket go a well, one day bottom gwine drop out."

Cramer sat quietly and allowed me to vent my frustrations for a while and then said, "No ebery day a Krismas."

Those Jamaican pearls of wisdom got a smile out of me. I fought hard not to smile, but I couldn't hold back.

She continued, "Let me tell you about patients I had who stopped trying. I watched patients who had given up and sat in their wheelchairs or lay in bed, dying both mentally and physically. One was a former professional football player I had on my ward who thought his illness was hopeless, so he gave up. Lying in bed one day, he turned his face to the wall and refused all nourishment and treatment. He died soon after. I believe he willed himself to die.

"On the other hand, I had patients who went to PT everyday, maintained hope, and made good progress. Some recovered completely."

I thought about what Rosa had told me about not showing nurses that I had given up. Showing a lack of spirit might cause them to give up on me too. I didn't want my lack of motivation to rub off on those from whom I needed help. I had seen it happen in the gym when therapists lost their enthusiasm to exercise patients who weren't motivated.

I noticed my thoughts about the "dry well" had become a trigger for slipping into feeling sorry for myself. It was clear that repeating those words and a few others had a powerful effect on my emotions. I knew I had to be more careful about using certain words and expressions that automatically triggered dark thoughts. Those words had become cues I had created through negative associations—exactly the opposite of the positive affirmations I should have been using.

I worried at times that my despondent moods might harm Cramer. I could be persuasive in my pessimistic outpourings and I worried I might bring her down with me. It would have been so easy for Cramer to join me in a "folie a deux" in which we fed off each others' negativity and both spiraled downward.

Thankfully, she never allowed herself to participate in my moods. When I was engaged in self-pity, she didn't buy into it. She empathetically stayed outside my mood and refused to allow herself to be drawn in. All the while I was spewing out negative thoughts, I was inwardly hoping she would counter my negativity with positive words. At the very time that I was telling her my situation was dire, another part of my mind was hoping she wouldn't be influenced and would keep reassuring me.

What would I have done if Cramer had agreed with me? and said, "Yes, Mr. Sweeta, I see what you're saying, you have good reason to be depressed. Your chances for improvement are poor."

I'm glad she never let down. Her wise counseling stimulated my rational prefrontal cortex and I felt more balanced.

On the other hand, Dr. Strak didn't help my peace of mind with his constant attempts to attach a psychological label on the cause of my paralysis, similar to the way doctors had put a physical label on my condition. Once doctors labeled it Guillain Barré Syndrome, it gave the false impression that it had been diagnosed and explained. However, the label was merely a name for a collection of symptoms. It didn't explain the causation or prescribe a treatment. Strak's psychological labeling would serve no better purpose.

In spite of his annoying ways, I got some pleasure from sparring with him. We had a kind of love-hate relationship. I was sure Dr. Strak didn't appreciate my opposition to his theories but he needed the hours of practicum to get his license, so he came by for our weekly session of give-and-take. In a strange way, I think he enjoyed the mental cat-and-mouse game we played with each other as much as I did. I wasn't sure who was the cat and who was the mouse—though his voice often had a high-pitched squeak.

During our sessions, Dr. Strak never stopped probing. He was a typical young psychologist, full of himself, believing his training was scientific rather than theoretical. He had to believe that to justify all the time and effort he had invested. He was caught up in the latest jargon and tried to impress me with his psycho-babble.

I asked Strak what method of therapy he practiced. He said he followed a bio-psycho-social model—which I saw as a way of putting pieces of different theories together and giving them a scientific sounding name. I asked him to explain.

He answered, "I've developed a method of therapy that combines the best information from biology, psychology, and sociology. It's a cross-discipline approach."

I smiled, "In other words, you've created a therapy to suit your personal beliefs."

Strak replied, "I guess you could say that."

I felt like sparring with him so I gave him a left jab, "But, in order to select what you believe are the best parts of all the available theories, you'd have to be knowledgeable in the hundreds of different theories, wouldn't you?"

He paused for a moment before jabbing back, "Well... no one could possibly be familiar with *every* theory out there."

I hit him with a right cross, "Then how can you be sure what you've selected from only a few is the best possible therapy?"

In defense, he countered, "I do what works best for me."

I sensed his growing agitation, so I jabbed again, "Dr. Strak, most of the therapies have radically different methods. They can't all be effective, can they?"

He answered in a high-pitched tone, "I think they all have their place in the system."

I sparred some more, "What system is that? Therapists don't follow one common, proven system. They use all kinds of methods which often conflict with one another. The confusing terminology makes them sound scientific—even a bit mystical."

Strak was now completely off balance and his voice was getting squeakier, "We need different types of therapies to handle different types of people with different types of problems. One size doesn't fit all."

That was a clever counter-punch, but I couldn't let him get off the ropes that easily, "That sounds good, Dr. Strak, but who matches patients with the so-called 'right' therapy? There isn't a system for doing that. Psychologists are free to practice whatever method they want—even if it's wacky. Right?"

Strak was still counterpunching, "I think the diversity of psychology is great. It allows us to be free-thinking and creative."

I countered, "But, that's the problem. The number of therapies keeps multiplying and today we've got more screwy therapies than we have screwy weight-loss diets. Today those diverse paths are so disconnected that all the king's horses and all the king's men couldn't put them back together again."

Strak was still punching back. He interrupted my little flurry, "It's necessary to go in different directions before you can find the right path. Thomas Edison went off in hundreds of wrong directions before he created the lightbulb. Psychology is trying to find the bulb that lights the way."

I couldn't let his cute analogy go uncontested, "Sure, Edison went down many wrong paths, but when he saw they didn't lead to an answer, he dumped them. Psychology doesn't do that. It keeps them all."

Like a bulldog, Strak wasn't going down without a fight, "I still say it's only a matter of time until our research finds the answers." He clung tenaciously to his belief that psychology was an exact science.

I went for the knockout, "Dr. Strak, psychologists love to do research on small pieces of human behavior, but they never connect the dots. Someone once said, 'The studies of smaller and smaller pieces of human behavior will lead us to know more and more about less and less until we know everything about nothing.' Psychologists can make bricks but they can't figure out how to put them together to build something useful."

After my analogy, there was dead silence. I had said all I wanted to say and Strak had heard all he wanted to hear. Dr. Strak had fought well, but I sensed he was a bit stunned as he left the arena to find some other patient who was more appreciative of his theories.

Strak had aroused my curiosity, so I wheeled myself to the hospital library to check on how many psychotherapies were presently being used. I didn't realize how muddy the field had become. They ranged all the way from Freud's emphasis on the mind's inborn drives and compulsions to Skinner's rejection of the concept of mind altogether and dealt only with conditioned behavior.

It seemed obvious to me that if any one of the hundreds of so-called "therapies" had proven effective, it would have nullified the rest. Psychotherapists gave the impression that a common body of knowledge underlaid all of the various therapies and that a basically singular method was used by all therapists--but it wasn't true. There was no consensus of opinion regarding the efficacy of one method of therapy over another as the best way to achieve results.

My eyes were getting tired from all the reading, so I closed the books and wheeled myself back to my room. I'd had enough mental exercise for one day.

Meanwhile, on the physical side, by following my exercise program, my condition had improved to the point I could sit in my wheelchair all day and walk long distances on my walker.

Both Mrs. Hunt and Mrs. Agard had offered to take me for a drive in their cars and spend a few hours outside the hospital. I was flattered by their offers, but I had politely refused.

I had reasons for not wanting to venture outside the hospital. My daily routine in the hospital was established and I didn't want to upset it. It was familiar to me. I had adapted to my routine. If I went out into the real world, I was concerned I might slip out of the mental groove I was in. Furthermore, I didn't want to be upset by seeing all the things I was missing.

Those thoughts rattled around in my brain. Besides, why do it now? Maybe it wouldn't be long before I'd be better and not have to worry about all those problems.

Or maybe I was just making excuses because I had become institutionalized....

Chapter 23

Who am I?

"These troublesome disguises which we wear..."
Paradise Lost, John Milton (1608-1674)

One afternoon, Hugh brought me a large cardboard box filled with all the mail I had accumulated during the time I was in the hospital. He had been saving it until the time when he thought I could deal with it.

Mrs. Agard patiently opened the hundreds of envelopes and handed the contents to me.

Most of my mail was junk mail, but there were many receipts relevant to the income tax filings I hadn't made for the past years. Whenever I left the hospital, I'd be faced with filing for those years and I didn't know whether the IRS would penalize me. It was just another problem I had to add to all my other problems of returning to life outside the hospital.

Meanwhile, I knew I couldn't avoid venturing out of the hospital indefinitely. There were too many opportunities and I was running out of excuses.

During one of our daily talks, Cramer asked me if I'd be interested in going on a hospital sponsored, deep-sea fishing trip. It sounded like fun, but I still didn't want to leave the security of the hospital. I didn't know what to say to her. She explained at length that there would be nurses going along to take care of the patients. It took a lot of convincing on her part, but she finally coaxed me into saying a reluctant "O.K."

Before I could change my mind, Cramer got on the phone and made the arrangements. It would be my first time away from the hospital.

Two days later, after breakfast, Cramer helped me get warmly dressed for the trip. I had mixed feelings. I thought it might be fun, but leaving the hospital was scary.

As I left the ward, Cramer said, "Walk good mon."

Eleven other patients and three accompanying nurses were loaded into the hospital van and driven to Los Angeles Harbor. The van didn't have windows in the rear area, so I couldn't see much of the outside world until we arrived at the San Pedro boat slip. The nurses wheeled us out of the van and up a ramp to board a large fishing boat.

We were soon underway, heading out into the vast Pacific Ocean. I sat by the railing near the bow and let my senses take in the panorama of sights, sounds, and smells. I watched the sailboats cruising through the gentle swells, listened to the gulls cruising overhead, and breathed in the tangy sea air.

I couldn't use my arms well enough to fish, but I enjoyed watching the others catch dozens of halibut and sea bass. At noontime, a nurse unwrapped the large hamburger the hospital had sent along for my lunch and she held it for me to eat. We spent the whole day on the water and got back to the hospital in time for the caught fish to be fried for our evening meal. I had thoroughly enjoyed my first trip outside the hospital and my face had a healthy glow from a combination of sun and wind. I was glad I went, but it took a while to mentally readjust to hospital life.

A few days later, Cramer told me the Patient Activities Office had tickets to a Dodger-Giants baseball game being played the next day. At first I wasn't interested, but the more I thought about it, the more I wanted to go. I had been outside the hospital on the fishing trip, but this was different. On the fishing boat, I only came in contact with a few of the boat's crew, but this time I'd be in the presence of forty thousand cheering baseball fans. That was a whole different situation. I had some doubts about going, but I had gained courage from the fishing trip and decided to take the step. I wheeled myself to the office and signed up.

The next day, eleven patients and three nurses were loaded into the hospital van and headed for Dodger Stadium. We drove down the freeway and soon arrived at the stadium parking lot. In the stadium, we had a space reserved for our wheelchairs behind the seats on the second deck.

During the game, a nurse asked me what I wanted from the foodstand. This was my chance for the chilidog I had been craving since my first day in the hospital. I almost shouted, "I want a chilidog with everything on it!"

After she left, I waited in anticipation of getting my beloved chilidog at long last.

Unfortunately, when the nurse returned, she said they didn't have chili or onions. It was just a plain hotdog with mustard. It wasn't the same. My long-awaited dream of a chilidog would have to wait for another time.

Caught up in the excitement of the game, my thoughts were transported to a time before hospitals and doctors and nurses. I was the old me watching the Dodgers fight it out with the Giants.

When the last out was made, my thoughts returned to reality. On the way back to the hospital, I felt troubled. The fishing trip and the Dodger ballgame were my first ventures outside the hospital. Until then, I had been sheltered inside the hospital and had completely adapted to my role as a patient. The two outings had allowed me to feel normal again for a while, but now I had to face returning to the hospital and once again reidentify myself as a patient.

Who the heck was I? My self-image shifted back and forth from being a patient, to being a normal person, and back to being a patient. Where did I belong? I wasn't sure.

My self-image confusion became more evident when Hugh visited me the next day.

"Hi John. I've been holding on to your keys for you, but you may as well have them."

He placed the keyring on the nightstand.

I looked at the keys and couldn't stop staring at them. I hadn't seen the keys in over two years. They seemed surreal. The sight of my car and house keys disturbed me and I didn't know why.

Later, after Hugh had left, I thought about why the sight of my keys had unnerved me. It was clear. Those keys were a direct, tangible connection to a past life that I had almost entirely shut out of my mind.

In order to make my life bearable in the hospital, I had not allowed myself to think too much about the outside world because it made me despondent. I knew if I dwelled on my former life, the long days in the hospital would be more difficult, so I built a mental wall between the two worlds. It happened very slowly, one thought at a time. The separation allowed me to adjust to my hospital life, but it also made me adopt the role of a patient. After two long years in the hospital,

I had become institutionalized in many ways without realizing it.

I had to be constantly alert because that mindset told me I couldn't do things for myself and had to be careful not to ask nurses to help me when it wasn't necessary.

I remembered reading about college students who spent a week in a retirement home with old people. After a few days, the young students began to talk and act like the old folks. The students became lethargic, stood less erect, and talked slower, with less enthusiasm. They had adapted to their environment by imitating the behavior they unconsciously believed was expected of them.

Looking at the other patients on the ward, I saw how the longer hospitalized ones had also adopted the behavior of their environment. They had acquired a "learned helplessness" and wanted nurses to help them eat, dress, toilet, and do other simple tasks. Some enjoyed the attention, some were plain lazy, and some had become psychologically dependent. They became like little boys and the nurses became their surrogate mothers. Some actually needed the assistance, but many could have done more for themselves if their dependency had not become a way of life. Once they had the self-image of a helpless patient, they stopped doing many things for themselves.

It was an easy trap to fall into for both patients and nurses. The patients enjoyed having everything done for them and many nurses felt it was easier to help them than to spend time and effort training them.

Mrs. Cramer knew the difference between helping and coddling a patient. Training patients was a challenge she enjoyed. She knew in the long run it would not only save herself time and trouble if patients were more independent, but the patients would benefit by becoming more active and self-confident.

Cramer never tried to hold on to her patients any more than she did her children. Being fiercely independent herself, she wanted others to be independent too. She often told me how she had given her children the freedom to be their own persons. If they needed her, she was there, but if they could do something for themselves, she stood aside. She believed in letting go. It wasn't something she read in a book, she instinctively knew.

We discussed how many parents tried to hold on to their children long after their children had become adults. Instead of developing an adult-to-adult relationship, they wanted to keep an adult-to-child relationship. The parents didn't want to lose the feeling of being needed.

Cramer believed a nurse's desire to be helpful shouldn't interfere with the patient's need to learn new skills. Anything less resulted in an unhealthy relationship that kept both parties from growing. She explained it was difficult at times to stand back and watch a patient struggle to button his pajamas or try to feed himself, but it was necessary. Otherwise, a patient would not progress and would remain dependent.

As my skills gradually improved, I depended less and less on Cramer. In the beginning, she did every little thing for me. However, one by one, she guided me to do things for myself.

Sometimes I looked into her eyes or listened to her voice, to see if I could detect a sign of regret because I didn't need her as much as I used to. I never saw it nor heard it. Instead, she kept pushing me to go farther. She got her joy from my independence, not my dependence. She knew that ultimately I might be independent enough to go home and our close relationship would be severed, but that didn't stop her. Cramer knew how to let go.

Even so, no matter how much she encouraged patients' independence, she was always there if they really needed help. Her credo was, "Never do for patients what they can do for themselves, and if they manage to do something once, they'll do it even better the next time."

One day I heard her admonish a nursing aide for starting to help a patient put on his pajamas. She told him to let the patient do it for himself. After a brief struggle, the patient managed to dress himself and beamed with pride for his accomplishment. The nursing aide was also proud that his patient had achieved a new skill.

Cramer admitted to me, "Sometimes, I feel I may be pushing patients a little too hard, but as long as I keep my expectations reachable, it all works out. It's exciting to see them try to meet my expectations once I establish a rapport with them. Patients try very hard not to disappoint nurses they have come to respect."

I was slowly becoming more independent, but many things were still hard to accomplish. I was attempting to learn how to walk with a quad-cane in the gym, but each step was a struggle. I had poor balance and couldn't walk more than twenty steps before I began trembling and sweating. The walker was still my best way to get around.

Cramer weighed me each week. My weight was up to 160 pounds. All the gains were new muscle distributed throughout my body.

Doug monitored my progress in PT and often made suggestions to Rick. One morning, Doug asked me if I'd like to try electrotherapy. He explained that he would administer a low voltage shock to my arms and legs which might jolt the nerves into contracting the muscles.

I was game, so we tried it for a week. It was extremely painful because Doug had to keep increasing the voltage. Every shock felt like needles being jammed in me. However, no matter how much voltage he used, none of my muscles spasmed. Doug was a compassionate man and said he was discontinuing the treatment after he saw how I winced in pain every time he applied the electric shock without producing results. I sighed with relief.

On my way back to the ward, I decided I could use a little fresh air. I wheeled myself out the hospital's front door and saw that it was raining. I stopped under the large canopy protecting the entrance and I could feel the mist from the rain falling outside my protective cover. Thunder rolled and brief flashes of lightning lit up the sky. It was a mild Spring shower.

Hospital staff and visitors with umbrellas, sheets of plastic, or newspapers covering their heads, were scurrying to cars picking them up or from cars dropping them off. They were all unhappy with the downpour.

I sat in my wheelchair enjoying the cool mist that blew over me. My mind drifted back to my days in intensive care when I wished for this exact moment. When I lay in the carefully controlled environment of ICU with no feeling of weather, no temperature changes, and no fresh air, I wondered if I'd ever feel a drop of rain on my face again. I vowed to myself that if I did, I'd enjoy every minute of the cool drops falling on my face. Now was that time.

I slowly wheeled my chair toward the end of the canopy. The nearer I got to the end, the heavier the mist became. One final push and I was out in the rain.

Just as I had pictured in my mind so many times, I turned my face to the sky and let the droplets bathe my face. It felt fantastic. I must have looked like a fool to some of the people who were trying to avoid the very thing I was enjoying. I didn't give a damn what they thought. I just kept smiling with my face to the sky while the raindrops gradually soaked my hair and my pajamas. I noticed a few people saw my joy and smiled back at me. Maybe one day I might lose my appreciation for the beauty of rain, but for now, I enjoyed this moment in time.

After a wonderful ten minutes, I was soaked to the skin but I couldn't care less. I had just had one of the happiest times of my life.

It was time for dinner so I reluctantly wheeled myself back to the ward. When I got back, Cramer saw me coming down the hall. She took one look at my wet hair, soaked pajamas, and the stupid grin on my face and said, "Wat ya bringin we? Dat not eye-wata on ya. Don ya know dat lil canoo asta keep by de shore?"

That's all she said as she stripped off my wet clothes, dried me off, and put fresh pajamas on me. She understood perfectly. She always did.

After dinner, Cramer informed me that Murphy was leaving the hospital. He had asked to be discharged. He wanted to go home though he was still in a wheelchair and far from being rehabilitated. His eighty-year-old mother would have to care for him as best she could.

I went to his room and asked him why he wanted to leave.

Murphy answered, "I asked to be discharged because I'm in a room with three sick guys who moan in pain all night. I also feel like my life is being wasted. All I do all day is hang around the cafeteria looking for someone to talk to. In the gym, my therapist isn't helping me that much, so I have to work out by myself. Heck, I can do that at home."

I advised, "Why don't you insist that your therapist help you more? You can go home when you're able to walk better."

"No, I want to go home now. I've been here for over two years. It's time to go."

I tried to talk him into staying, but he had made up his mind. I understood his wanting to go home.

Murphy looked sad as he said, "What did I do wrong for God to do this to me? I always treated people well. I go to church every Sunday?"

I had heard the same lament from other patients. It seemed many patients had this same idea that God was punishing them because they had committed some terrible sin. People were always feeling guilty about something or another and illness gave them a perfect outlet.

I tried to comfort Murphy by saying, "Murphy, you didn't do anything wrong. God isn't some cruel power that waits for you to do something wrong so he can punish you."

I followed, "The way I see it, God sometimes challenges you. Think of it as his way of testing your belief—like right now. Each time you keep the faith, you get spiritually stronger. Stop blaming yourself Murphy. Your illness has nothing to do with having offended God."

I had Murphy thinking.

As I wheeled away, I was also concerned that if he left, I was losing my buffer. Since Murphy had Guillain Barré too and was in better shape than I was, I knew they wouldn't discharge me before him. But, with his leaving, I was probably next on the list to be discharged. Since I wasn't as functional as Murphy, I would probably be sent to a nursing home. I had no place else to go. I needed a lot of daily assistance and there was no one to take care of me. The thought of going to a nursing home was unsettling.

I had been carefully monitoring my improvements and the results were discouraging. In the last two months, my progress had slowed to an imperceptible level. My legs were still weak and I saw no improvement in walking with a cane. It was difficult to use and falling could be disastrous. Rick and I agreed I should go back to using the walker.

Occupational therapy for my hands had also hit a wall. There was nothing more Judy could do to help. She had massaged my hands as best she could and the knuckles remained frozen. I stopped my appointments.

The longer I stayed in the hospital, the more disappointed I became with my slow progress. Exercising every day had taken its toll on me. After two long years of physical therapy, I was a million miles away from being independent enough to make a life for myself outside the hospital.

My dream of a "sharp corner" recovery had been over for a long time. The miracle hadn't happened and it wasn't going to. What I needed was to return to a longterm attitude, a steady paced, even flow of positive thinking with realistic, short-term goals. I would simply be allowing things to happen in their own time—going with the flow. That would ease the frustrations and keep my feelings in balance.

Mrs. Hunt once told me, "John, your progress will be like watching grass grow. You can't see it happening, but with patience you'll notice the difference after a while." She was probably right.

My visitors from Alcoholics Anonymous said they believed that letting go of the conscious struggle against life's misfortunes, tapped into a "higher power." They said the second step of their recovery process was to gracefully surrender to a power greater than themselves. It could be a supreme being or simply some universal energy—just connect to *whatever* the hell it is.

Some psychiatrists believed the mere act of "letting go" released a healing energy. Letting the subconscious mind take control eliminated conscious doubts while it subliminally worked on the problem.

Chapter 24

Troubling Thoughts

"God, give us grace to accept with serenity the
things that cannot be changed, courage to
change the things which should be changed, and
the wisdom to distinguish the one from the other."
Reinhold Neibuhr, The Serenity Prayer

I found that letting go had a calming effect on me. I saw
things more clearly when the pressure from expecting too
much from myself was relieved. It gave me the sense to know
the difference between things I could change and things I had
to accept, knowing when to fight and when to ease up. It was a
welcome relief.

Whenever I became discouraged, I'd take a day off and do
nothing. When I resumed my usual routine, I noticed I enjoyed
exercising more and was stronger than before.

One day while waiting for Rick to finish working with his
cardiac patient on the treadmill, I happened to be sitting next
to a rack with steel dumbbells. They ranged from a tiny two-
pound weight to an ominous looking twenty-five pounder.
Having nothing better to do, I reached over and picked up the
little two-pound dumbbell. As small as it was, I still had to
struggle to wrestle it into my lap because my hands couldn't
grip it properly. The tiny steel weight felt good in my hands. It
was like a link to my past when I was healthy and strong.

I held the weight with both hands and did a few simple
curls. It wasn't much, but it was a start. It was the beginning of
my renewed connection with weightlifting. I was so joyful to be
weightlifting again that I kissed the cool steel.

In the following days, I increased the size of the dumbbell
for curling. First the two-pounder, then the five-pounder, then
the ten. The weight might not be heavy for a normal person,
but it was huge for someone like me who hadn't used his
biceps in over two years. Just to hold that weight and do
something with it felt great. I was smiling and happy as I
moved the weight up and down. What a joy it was to feel my

muscles stretching, flexing, and responding to the weight's resistance. It brought back wonderful memories.

I had exercised all my life, so working with weights in the gym was like visiting old friends. After so many months of not being able to use my arms at all, I took a lot of pleasure in my ability to lift weights and use the pulley machine. My arm strength improved slightly each week.

The gym had a flight of five wooden stairs with a landing at the top that was designed for patients to practice climbing. My right leg was stronger than my left, so I was able to steady myself on the railings with both hands and slowly lift my right foot onto the next step and push myself up, one stair at a time till I reached the top landing. I descended by backing down in reverse order. It was an important skill I would need in the real world.

In my room, I was now able to transfer myself in and out of bed. To get out of bed, I electrically elevated the head of my bed to a sitting position, then swung my legs out onto the floor and got on my walker. I reversed the order to get back in bed.

It was also time for me to start showering myself. There was no reason to depend on Cramer anymore for that. As I wheeled myself down the hall, Cramer asked me where I was going.

I replied, "To shower."

She smiled and nodded her approval.

I was able to transfer to the shower chair, turn on the water, and apply soap to all the right places. Another milestone.

My exercise plan of letting things happen in their own time was working well. I had been following my exercise plan and was making some progress without any negative effects, so I accelerated my workouts. I slouched down and did partial sit-ups in my wheelchair till my stomach muscles burned. I walked all around the second floor on my walker, timing my trip and trying to make the circuit faster each day. Throughout the day, I exercised my hands at every opportunity.

I was enjoying exercising more than ever. To keep my motivation high, I visualized myself as an athlete in training with my muscles growing stronger and stronger. My mind felt in balance.

Now, I had a greater range of motion and I could work some muscles to their limit using weights. I had reached a higher level of exercising. Soreness and stiffness resulted. Was I overdoing it? Was I allowing enough time between exercises for my muscle tissue to regenerate? If not, I could be retarding my progress or even causing harm. I didn't know whether to continue exercising daily and risk overstressing my muscles, or to change my routine and cut back, which could possibly delay my progress. I wasn't sure which way was best. I had to think it through.

I sat back and drew upon my many years of exercise experience. Professional bodybuilders exercised every day, but they alternated using different areas of the body. One day upper body, next day lower body. I remembered reading a study of marathon runners which found that runners who took time off between heavy running in order to let their muscles recuperate, progressed better than runners who kept working the same muscles daily. I had noticed in the past that I was stronger after resting my exercised muscles for a day.

I came up with a plan. I'd continue exercising every day. However, I wouldn't exercise the same muscle group every day. One day I'd exercise legs, next day arms and chest.

In the gym, I could now take a few steps between the parallel bars without using my hands for support. I grabbed onto the bars quickly when I lost my balance.

Rick saw my success walking between the bars, so he prepared me to walk outside the bars while he held onto a safety belt. He strapped the belt around my chest and he was there to catch me if I started to topple over. I was prepared to take that first solo step.

I stepped forward with my stronger right leg. It felt unsteady, but to keep my balance I had to keep moving. I followed that first step quickly with my left leg. I knew if I stopped, I'd fall. Right, left, wobble, right, left, oops, right, left— I made it to a chair. My first solo flight! It was a fearful, ungraceful, wobbly walking, but it was real walking. For the first time in over two years, I had taken steps without any help. My adrenalin was pumping and I felt a wonderful high.

But, trying to walk without Rick was different because I had a tremendous fear of falling. Normally, people could break their fall and cushion the impact, but if I fell, my full weight would hit the floor. A broken leg or hip at this time would be devastating. It would set my walking back to square one.

After a few weeks of walking with Rick, I was able to walk a little farther. However, I never felt secure or steady and there was the constant fear of falling.

In my room, one evening, I felt confident enough to try walking from my wheelchair to the bathroom without anyone nearby to assist me. I flipped up the footrests, pushed myself up, and stood for a moment, holding on to the wheelchair's armrests until I felt steady. I let go of the wheelchair and took a bold step.

I immediately began to fall. It felt like it was happening in slow motion. I actually fell in one quick plunge to the floor, but mentally, it seemed to happen in stages, like a stop-action film. In the first stage, I thought "Oh no" when I realized I was falling. In stage two, I felt the pain in my knees as they bent under the weight of my collapsing body. The third stage was my buttocks hitting the floor, then my back, and finally my head as it flopped backward and hit with a thud.

I lay there quietly, checking my body to see if I was hurt. My toes hurt badly from the extreme bending forward and my buttocks were aching, but otherwise I wasn't cut or injured. My head lay between the flipped-up steel footrests of the wheelchair. If my head had hit one of them, I would have been seriously injured. I had been extremely lucky.

I yelled for help. Mrs. Agard and Mrs. Hunt came running and lifted me back into the wheelchair. They asked me if I was hurt and gave me a thorough check to make sure I was all right. Except for sore toes and buttocks, I felt okay.

The incident showed me I was in no condition to try walking by myself. Though my legs were strong enough, the nerves below my ankles had not regenerated, so I couldn't move any muscles in my feet to make the precise balancing corrections that toe and foot muscles normally make. If I was ever to walk without using a walker, those nerves would have to return—and with each passing month, the chances grew slimmer. I had to accept the possibility that I might have to use the walker indefinitely.

I was still a bit sore the next morning, but forgot about it in the bustle of activity on the ward. Every few months, a class of nursing students from a local college came on the ward as part of their practical training. They did basic bedside nursing to get real-life experience. Cramer and her staff appreciated the extra hands. Once in a while, she permitted students to care for me under her supervision.

After a few classes had come through, I got to know Meredith, the dean of the school. She accompanied the students to monitor their progress. One afternoon, Meredith asked me if I'd be interested in giving a seminar to the student nurses and share my insights and experiences as a patient. I happily accepted her offer. She asked Cramer to co-host.

The following week, Cramer and I held the seminar in a hospital classroom. I described my paralysis to the student nurses and explained in detail my difficult, slow stages of recovery, both physical and mental. Cramer's explanation from a nurse's point of view offered an interesting contrast. The students' questions afterward reflected they had acquired useful information for their future work as nurses.

The seminar went so well that Cramer and I were asked to give a seminar to the following class. Meredith believed the two-way discussions helped students learn about the psychological aspects of nursing.

After the second seminar, Meredith asked me to consider giving the commencement speech to her next graduating class. I didn't hesitate in accepting her offer. Nurses were my favorite people.

Besides my life as a patient, I also had a social life in the hospital as I interacted with nurses, doctors, therapists, visitors, and other patients. The ward had a dayroom where patients could sit around and read, play games, and get to know each other. Once a month, a man and his wife visited our ward and brought homemade cookies and refreshments for us to enjoy while she sang to her husband's accompaniment on the piano. It was always a pleasant afternoon of music, good food, and warm interaction. I tried not to think about the likelihood I would never again play the piano—a bitter loss.

But, was it a total loss? I could still wiggle my fingers even though I couldn't actually control them. I wondered whether I could press a couple of piano keys and somehow play a song, so one day I wheeled myself into the dayroom and sat in front the piano.

I played the melody line of a song I knew by using the index finger of my right hand. I thought, "Hey, I'm making music." So, I tried using my thumb to press two notes away from my index finger to make harmony. "Not too bad," I thought. That was as much as I could do with my right hand.

What about my left hand? It was less usable, but I could use my left index finger to play one note at a time on the lower, bass keys.

It only took three notes to form a chord so I played some two-handed, three-fingered chords. More importantly, I could play a chord with only my left index finger by quickly rolling the three notes of a chord to the accompaniment of my right hand's melody. It worked like magic!

It was only a matter of time and practice until I could play songs that sounded quite good. I amazed myself at the quality I achieved by using my musical background and a little ingenuity. I definitely was playing music that sounded good and not like someone fumbling around on the piano. I sometimes played for my visitors, who were also amazed at how well it sounded. I was sure I was the best three-fingered piano player this side of the Mississippi. It was another example of what I could do if I tried. Regaining my ability to create music again breathed new life into me and added to my renaissance.

The hospital didn't have rigid visiting hours. I wished it had. I welcomed visitors except when they interfered with my daily routine or stayed too long. It was nice to have people drop in to chat and offer their support, but sometimes they disturbed my schedule. One visitor came when I was about to be wheeled outside on the patio to sunbathe and enjoy my daily afternoon nap. He stayed for an hour, canceling out my nap. I didn't want to seem ungrateful to people taking time out of their own busy lives to visit me, but with no strictly enforced visiting hours, people came at lunchtime, dinnertime, therapy time, and late in the day when I needed to get to bed.

Living in my small room was like living in a fishbowl; the door was always open and I was on view to everyone who passed by. If they felt like talking, they walked right in. That included visitors from outside the hospital as well as patients and staff inside the hospital. People seemed to be coming and going at all hours.

One problem with having so many people drifting in and out was theft. It was unfortunate that in a hospital, there were people who stole from patients, but it happened. I had bought an expensive watch from the hospital canteen and kept it in my nightstand drawer. One morning, I saw it was missing when I opened the drawer. There were so many people entering my room everyday that I had no idea who had taken it. I was positive it wasn't one of the nurses.

Another theft occurred a few days later. I always kept some cash in the pack hanging on the back of my wheelchair. One day, when I looked in the pack, I noticed the eighty dollars I had had there was gone. Someone had stealthily gone into my pack during the day while I was sitting in the wheelchair and stolen the money.

Until those two thefts, it had never occurred to me that anyone would steal from helpless patients. Now I knew better and was more cautious.

I wondered how all the people entering my room would appreciate having the front door of their homes always open and people coming in at all hours. All I wanted was a little privacy.

Some visitors were a problem because they didn't know how long to stay. The "visitors dilemma" was they didn't know if they were staying too long or not staying long enough. The ideal visitor for me was someone who prepared to leave after about fifteen minutes and then waited for me to ask them to stay longer if I felt like spending more time with them. For most visitors, the conversations usually became uncomfortable and forced after about fifteen minutes.

There were times when I desperately wished I had visitors because I was lonely and needed someone to talk to. But, there were times when I just wanted to be left alone to rest. Most visitors were wonderful people whom I really enjoyed seeing. But, even they could overstay their welcome if they didn't use a little common sense. Some stayed for an hour or more and were oblivious to my body language telling them it was time to leave. They didn't pick up on my cues when I stopped responding to them or kept turning my eyes away to watch TV. Some people simply didn't know how to end a conversation and say goodbye.

One visitor came when I was already in bed and droned on talking for an hour even after I closed my eyes to sleep.

Visitors came in all types. Most came to genuinely offer their support. A few came for their own personal reasons. One visitor was a religious fanatic and came to preach the word of God to me. I patiently listened to his long sermons of how my illness was part of God's plan and how God had a wonderful cure planned for me.

Other visitors enjoyed visiting to tell me about their own previous illnesses, explaining in depth their painful operations. I certainly wasn't interested in hearing all that.

Another problem with some of my visitors was they wanted me to explain in detail how my recovery was coming along. It was nice of them to be interested in my progress, but when they wanted to examine every little detail of my condition, it became mentally fatiguing and forced me to focus on the negative things that I'd rather not dwell on. If I simply answered, "Fine" or "Okay," they often continued probing and left me feeling dejected after having forced me to explain my problems in detail. I wished visitors asked only general questions and let me decide whether or not to go into detail, rather than interrogating me.

It was frustrating when visitors asked me to show my progress by moving parts of my body I couldn't move. They meant well, but I wished they hadn't insisted. I felt like a performing animal in a show when I went through my routine of demonstrating my limited hand and leg movements.

A typical request was, "Let's see you make a fist." I tried and always failed.

They insisted, "You're not trying hard enough. I know you can do it."

So I tried over and over without success. I wanted to please them, but I couldn't. Every attempt was a reminder of my dysfunction and reinforced my feelings of helplessness. All

I was doing was frustrating myself and disappointing them. When I failed, I felt like a fool.

Finally, I had to say, "I can't do it."

Sometimes they persisted, "How do you know you can't do it? Try again."

Did they think I hadn't previously tried to do it on my own? I had to remind myself that none of them realized I had gone through this routine dozens of times before with others. For each of them, it was a new experience. I didn't want them to have an unpleasant visit, so I put on a happy face and tried to keep the conversation lighthearted. I felt obligated to cheer *them* up.

There were always moments of awkward silence when visitors didn't know what to say. Feeling uncomfortable, they usually tried to fill the void with trivialities, not understanding that silences were meaningful and important and didn't need to be filled in with words. They didn't understand that all they had to do was relax and be themselves.

After months of hospitalization, I longed for human touch other than nurses' handling. I had read about lonely people who got massages or had their nails done or their hair cut just to be touched by another human being. I appreciated a visitor's hug or handclasp.

Being a good visitor was a skill—and so was being a good host to visitors. We learned from each other as we went along.

Since my friend Murphy had left, I believed I would be discharged soon. I'd been in the hospital for two and a half years. Time was against my staying. The hospital was not a warehouse, so the only ones who stayed were those too ill to be sent to a nursing home. I was a prime candidate for discharge since my vital signs were stable and I was almost self-care. The only thing keeping me in the hospital was my physical therapy. As long as the doctors thought I was benefiting from PT, they might allow me to stay, but once they saw I was physically able, it would be a signal to send me to a nursing home. I saw patients in worse shape than me sent to nursing homes. The rationale for transferring patients was the unlikelihood of further significant improvement.

In spite of potential discharge, I never stopped trying to do things for myself. Each week I accomplished a little more. One day, I managed to wiggle myself into my pajama bottoms and slip on the tops. Soon thereafter, I was able to pull on my socks. Another day, my shoes. My ability to put on clothes was a meaningful achievement. I had reached a new level of independence. The ability to get in and out of bed, dress myself, feed myself, and get around on the walker meant I could function independently *outside* the hospital!

However, I wasn't ready to leave the hospital yet because I believed I could improve even more with continued physical therapy.

The quandary of whether to stay or leave was settled for me when Charlene visited. She told me that Chris hadn't been doing well in highschool ever since I'd been in the hospital and I should seriously consider coming home because he needed the strong influence of a father. If I did come home, she wanted to know if I'd be willing to have him live with me so I could give him the full-time guidance she wasn't able to.

I wasn't through with my physical rehabilitation, but I believed it was more important to take care of Chris, so I said I would do it. My hospitalization had already caused too much damage to both my life and his. However, I told Charlene I couldn't leave the hospital until I found a job to support Chris and me when I left the hospital.

I was in a Catch 22 situation. I wanted to improve my physical condition as much as possible before I left, but if I appeared too self-sufficient, the doctors might decide to discharge me before I found a way to earn a living. Without a job, I'd be financially unable to support myself and Chris. I would end up in a county nursing home and that wouldn't help Chris.

I decided the best plan was to keep a low profile. While I kept out of sight, I'd try to improve my walking, using my hands, and whatever other abilities I'd need in everyday living.

I knew one thing for sure, I couldn't stay much longer in the hospital and going to a nursing home wasn't an option I wanted to consider. I had to physically and mentally prepare myself for leaving the hospital and living on my own. A job was the crux of making it on the outside.

But, how could I get a job while still in the hospital? If a company responded to my mailed resumé, how could I get to an interview? Who would hire me in a wheelchair or on a walker? I had to come up with a plan for getting a job. It didn't look hopeful.

In a wonderful stroke of luck, the problem was solved when Tom Rauscher, one of my oldest friends, visited me. During his visit, we discussed my desire to go back to work. Tom said he'd talk to his engineering manager about the possibility of hiring me. I was hesitant about taking such a huge step, but Tom assured me the job required my brain, not my body. After a few encouraging words from him, I agreed to give it a try.

After he left, my mind was spinning with questions. "Have I lost my job skills? Will co-workers accept me in my handicapped condition? Can I survive in a normal world?"

I didn't have much time to talk myself out of it because Tom phoned the following day and said he had an interview set up on December 12th. That was only a few weeks away. Tom and my other old buddies had talked to the manager of their engineering department and said they had a friend who was being released from the hospital and needed a job. They highly recommended me so he agreed to give me an interview. Things were moving quickly—maybe too quickly.

I thought about the fact that life would be much more difficult on the outside. In the hospital, I was just another patient, but on the outside, I would be seen as a handicapped person who was "different." In the hospital, I was near the top of the patient ladder; but outside I'd be on the lowest rung. In the hospital, I had a support system of doctors and nurses and my disability was in an accepting environment. Outside the hospital's sheltering womb, my disability would be magnified in a world of normal people. Inside, no one looked at me with a mixture of pity and rejection; outside I'd probably be labeled "handicapped" or "crippled."

Those unpleasant thoughts made me want to work harder to prepare myself for the outside. I had been steadily gaining weight and was up to 170 pounds, but I couldn't expect to add any more muscle unless I was able to handle heavier weights in the gym and I was already straining myself.

Walking was a bigger problem. I wanted to walk better before I left. My greatest worry was that my knees would buckle. I didn't dare walk too boldly because of the risk of falling and injuring myself. That prevented me from pushing my walking exercises and greatly limited my progress. Since I didn't have the strength to break my fall, I'd fall hard. A broken leg would set me back months. A fractured hip or spinal injury might cause permanent damage and confine me to a wheelchair or bed for life. The risks were too great to push myself too far beyond my limits. The walker was still my best option.

In spite of all my worries and fears, I was starting to feel good about the idea of getting a job and going home.

The next morning, I felt in high spirits when I awoke to Cramer's voice saying "Good morning" to patients as she came down the hall. After my morning cleansings, I got ready for breakfast. The food service lady brought me my breakfast tray and I heartily ate the bacon and eggs and washed them down with hot black coffee. I was ready for a great day. Nothing was going to bother me today. I felt great.

After breakfast, I went to PT.

In the gym, I walked in the parallel bars by myself—but after a minute, for no apparent reason, I started to lose my motivation. I could feel myself becoming sluggish and a little depressed. I decided to stop exercising and I wheeled myself back to the ward.

I thought a little fresh air and sunshine might brighten my flagging spirits, so I wheeled myself out onto the patio. It didn't help. I still felt out of sorts. Maybe it was all due to my apprehension about my coming interview for a job.

During the rest of the day, I argued with people for no reason. I was having a meltdown. I seemed to enjoy my angry outbursts. It felt good to let off steam. No one was safe. I even spoke harshly to Cramer—which I hardly ever did.

By that evening, I had expelled most of my negative energy and was thinking more sensibly. I had vented my feelings and relieved the tension—thankfully without causing any serious problems. That had been the wrong way to regain my mental balance. I should not have cut my gym workout short and should have continued to burn off my negative energy. The fact that I felt the negative energy churning inside me was the very reason I should have continued to exercise, not stop. I knew better. I knew the rules for keeping myself balanced and that if I kept practicing them, it would get easier and easier to maintain the balance.

The next day, Cramer said with a smile, "The patient in the next room is acting a little crazy today too. He made a hat out of newspaper and insisted I turn the head of his bed to face north. He didn't explain why. He's a little weird, but I thought if it would make him feel more secure, I saw no harm in transfering him to a bed facing north. Now he's happy and the problem is solved."

Cramer continued, "I have another patient who was a colonel in the Army. This morning, he asked me if he could see General Eisenhower. Sometimes he addresses the nurses as lieutenants and captains. Except for these passing delusions, his thinking is fairly rational."

I couldn't help saying, "Everyone is irrational at times, even you and me. Millions of people smoke in spite of knowing the health risks. Look at all the people who believe they were abducted by aliens and had medical examinations performed on them. People believe they've lived previous lives and were once somebody famous. Millions of women watch soap operas and believe the stories are real. Just about everyone believes in either UFO's, fortune tellers, psychics, or ghosts. Our minds can create all kinds of illusions we swear are real."

I continued, "But, just because people believe in a few strange things doesn't mean they're nuts. Except for those few weird ideas, they lead regular lives. I believe everybody's mind shifts between rational and irrational thoughts all day long. No one has figured out the mysterious mazes inside the jelly between our ears, and I hope they never do."

Cramer interrupted, "So, who's crazy and who isn't?"

Wise old Mark Twain said, "When we remember we are all mad, the mysteries disappear and life stands explained. Sanity and happiness are an impossible combination."

I shrugged my shoulders, "I guess if you're somehow able to function in everyday life in spite of your weird ideas, you qualify to run loose."

What started out as a silly discussion about a patient wearing a paper hat, somehow had turned into a discussion of how strangely the human mind worked at times.

I laughed, "Mrs. Cramer, if your patient wants to wear a paper hat and have his bed face north, he's not crazy, he's just practicing Feng Shui. A billion Chinese can't be wrong."

Chapter 25

Burnout!

"Out, out, brief candle…"
MacBeth, William Shakespeare

After breakfast the next day, I noticed Mrs. Hunt hadn't been on duty for the past week. I asked Cramer where she was.

At first Mrs. Cramer avoided the question, but when she saw I wouldn't be put off, she answered briefly, "Mrs. Hunt has retired."

I was shocked. "What? I don't believe it! I talked with her every day and she never said anything to me about retiring."

Cramer sat down to explain, "Well, as I understand it, she's been under a lot of stress lately and she simply couldn't deal with it anymore. Mrs. Hunt was a very caring nurse and she gave too much of herself to her work.

"She's been taking care of her invalid mother at home in the evenings after working so hard here on the ward all day. You should understand as well as anyone how much care she gave to everyone—except herself. She simply burned out. A nurse can only give so much. At some point, there's nothing left to give."

I was stunned. "I still can't believe it. She had a master's degree and more than twenty years of experience. Didn't she know how to deal with her stress?"

Maryann was nearby listening to our conversation, so I asked her, "Maryann, I feel terrible about what happened to Mrs. Hunt. You're a psychiatric nurse. How could burnout happen to a great nurse like her? Didn't she realize that stress was getting the best of her?"

Maryann understood my question only too well. As a mental health nurse, she had seen the effects of stress on nurses more times than she wanted to remember.

"John, burnout has been called the 'occupational disease' of nurses. It seems to happen to the best nurses because they care so much and internalize too much. In a recent survey, half the nurses scored high for emotional exhaustion.

"Physically, the work is difficult and the responsibilities are immense. The pace is fast and the hours are long. Many nurses complain about doing too many non-nursing chores like foodtray handling, transporting patients, and paperwork. After a time, the mental and physical exhaustion from daily pressures and work overload can become overwhelming.

"John, I could go into a long explanation, but I have a better idea. There is a series of lectures on stress starting this Friday. If you're interested, I'd like you to attend. Maybe you'll understand a little more about the pressures that nurses have to deal with day after day. The first lecture will be this Friday evening in room 605 and you're welcome to attend. You might even get some good ideas to help you through your own tough times."

She didn't have to tell me twice, "I'll be there."

On Friday, I wheeled my chair into the conference room. It was a small room that held about fifty chairs. I rolled my wheelchair behind the last row and got my good old tape-recorder set up.

Before the lecture even began, it was standing room only. Stress was obviously a subject of great importance to nurses.

I attended all three lectures. The lecturer, Dr. Holmes, covered a lot of material and most of the information regarding stress applied to me and people in general. I would later incorporate many of these ideas in my overall plan to balance my inner energies. After the last lecture, I copied in my notebook the information from the tapes I recorded so I could refer to it later.

When I had finished, I sat back and reviewed my written notes...

Lecture 1: What Is Stress and Its Causes?

Scientific journals contain dozens of conflicting definitions of stress. Basically, there are two types of stress: known origin and unknown origin. Known origin stress is caused by a specific experience that is obvious, e.g. work pressures, money problems, spousal conflicts, etc.

Unknown origin stress is chronic, persistent and its cause is not readily identified. This may be due to deep pychological issues which require more intensive therapy to bring out the deep psychological origins. Unknown origin stress is a subject for a later time; today we are dealing with known origin stress.

Stress means different things to different people. Since we all experience some kind of stress daily, it's how we perceive and react to situations that makes the difference between stimuli we feel as either exciting or troubling.

One nurse's stress from a job seen as too demanding can be experienced by another nurse as exciting becaue the daily challenges keep her job interesting, like ER nurses. One nurse's stressful feellings from the pressures of an overload of work may not be felt the same way by another nurse who takes pride in organizing to get it all done, one thing at a time. The stress one nurse feels because her supervisor expects too much from her, may be experienced by another nurse as her supervisor's way of complimenting her ability to get things done by choosing her for the tough jobs. Stress is as stress is perceived.

Psychologists once believed everyone was seeking a stress-free state of mind. But, now we know people don't want to live a life of dull equilibrium. An environment with too little stimulation is also stressful. People crave stimulation. They need sensory input, not a bland state of mind. Some stress is a necessary and even a desirable part of living. Without the proper amount of stimulation, people will unconsciously create their own excitement by engaging in mental activities that are often irrational—as shown by sensory deprivation studies.

The problem occurs when we are overstimulated and the amount of stress is more than we can assimilate. We all have different thresholds, or tolerances, for handling stress and we try to keep our level balanced with our inborn tolerance to deal with it.

You don't need a psychologist to tell you when you're feeling too much stress. Your gut feelings will tell you. Humans need psychological stimulation—but not too much and not too little.

Lecture 2: What Are the Effects of Stress?

(a) Underlined Physical Effects: Stress causes wear and tear on the body. It turns physical when the body cannot maintain normal functioning due to changes in pulse rate, blood pressure, and other bodily rhythms. Stress disrupts the body's delicate balance of chemicals, namely (a) Dopamine, a morphine-like endorphin that acts as the body's painkiller and anti-depressant hormone, (b) Acetylcholine, a neurotransmitter that leads to depression if interfered with, (c) Cortisol, the chief stress fighting hormone, (d) Serotonin, which regulates the body's clock, and (e) Norepinephrine, which prepares the body for fight or flight. A person's reaction to stressors determines the type and amount of chemicals released or inhibited.

When the amount of endocrine secretions is altered, stress symptoms of insomnia, headaches, backaches, indigestion, night sweats, nervous twitching, or bursts of crying occur. It is nature's warning of more serious things to come.

If unchecked, stress can lead to serious disorders of the heart, metabolism, digestion, and resistance to infection.

(b) Psychological Effects: The first warning sign that stress is a problem is when you constantly feel tired and don't sleep well. Personal grooming becomes less important. The mind is filled with anxiety and feels like it's being squeezed in a vise. The anxiety affects your ability to think clearly and make good decisions. You're disorganized, confused, and not in control. Small problems are magnified. Everything is taken too seriously. There is a heaviness in your mind with thoughts of impending doom. You feel trapped and see no way out.

You know you need to change something because you can't continue this way, but you feel helpless to do anything about it. The pressures can expand like an inflated balloon and if the pressure reaches its bursting point, the mind will unload itself in uncontrollable bursts of emotion. It's nature's safety valve opening to release the tension.

If allowed to reach this point, it will take rest and psychological counseling to get the mind back on track again. But, unlike a burst balloon, the mind can restore itself. However, it's better to have ways to relieve pressures as they occur and not let them accumulate till the mind is forced to relieve itself in uncontrollable outbursts.

To prevent further harmful stress, the mind has the option of separating itself from reality until it finds a state of withdrawal that is tolerable. Denial is the mildest way of shutting out disturbing stimuli, wherein a person simply puts common sense aside and pretends the problem doesn't exist. Stressful stimuli may also be repressed by shoving problems into the subconscious. However, in the subconscious, they continue to accumulate and fester. Neither denial nor repression resolves the stress, they merely ignore its existence and give temporary relief. Sooner or later, the stress will cause problems and have to be dealt with.

Continuing stress that isn't relieved can lead to burnout. Burnout occurs when a person is drained physically and emotionally. When stress reaches that critical level, a person doesn't enjoy anything about her job and feels no one appreciates her efforts. She is irritated by little things co-workers do. She takes frequent sickdays and reaches a point where she feels the need to get away. Work stress carries over to homelife and disrupts family relationships.

Lecture 3: How To Deal with Stress in Sensible Ways
The first step in relieving stress is admitting to yourself you have a problem. Awareness is the first step. Pay attention to the changes in your body and mind. You can't ignore stress indefinitely. It won't go away by pretending everything is okay. You must realize that you need to do something before it becomes debilitating.

Basic things you can do to control stress:
The following is a list of practical suggestions for releasing the pressures of stress gradually. Select the ones that make the most sense to you. Start out with a few and add as you go along. Find the ones that work for you.

Start the day right. Don't think about your problems first thing in the morning. Things always look worse when you first wake up. Wait until you're dressed and had your morning coffee or breakfast and your mind is clear.

Reduce work hours till things are under control.

Minimize changes in your life and environment, postpone major changes.

Avoid people who are downers and sap your energy. Avoid people who make constant demands on you. Find people who support you and nourish you. Minimize social obligations by saying "no" when you really don't want to do something.

A support system of the right people is important. Everyone needs help at times. Talk to someone with whom you can express your deepest feelings: a family member, a friend, or a clergyman. If none of these things help, see a counselor or a psychologist to help clarify your problems so you can work things out.

Remember the importance of gratitude. Everyone has things in their life that are positive and good. Instead of always focusing on the negative, make a list of all the good things in your life and review the list whenever you're feeling down. Some psychologists believe that feelings of happiness are the result of feeling grateful.

Find words and ideas that motivate you and make you feel good. Practice saying those positive affirmations daily until the inspirational thoughts become a part of the inner you. Repetition is important to weld those ideas firmly in place.

Avoid thinking exaggerated thoughts like, "I'm losing my mind" or "Everything is hopeless." Keep your choice of words less extreme. Use specific, simple terms, not wild generalities.

When facing a stressful situation, ask yourself, "How important is this?" If it's not that important, stop anguishing over it. If you must worry, worry about something that's worth doing something about.

Give your hang-ups a rest. Make a specific time of day when you do nothing—no people, no telephone, no nothing. Sometimes doing nothing is the right thing.

You need not give all your energies to your family and put your own life on hold. You can't help others until you've helped yourself.

Have some fun. Let loose and be a kid again. Find humor in your life. Lighten up and laugh out loud, watch TV sitcoms, read the comic pages instead of the "news." Keep mentally handy a list of things that makes you smile when you think about them.

Take time out to read a light novel you've been putting aside. Read an inspiring self-help book like "Don't Sweat the Small Stuff." It can become a guideline for dealing with many of life's basic problems.

Re-visit the Bible, Talmud, or Quran and allow religion back into your life if you've been neglecting your faith. Let a higher-power help you get through the low times.

Find time to listen to soft, soothing music that relaxes you. Keep the rooms in your house bright with light.

Nutrition is important. Stabilize your blood sugar by eating frequent small meals instead of a few large meals. Constant thirst and excessive urination signal your blood sugar is too high. Irritability and excessive perspiration signal your sugar may be too low.

Enjoy simple pleasures. Plant some flowers. Look for beauty everywhere. Drive to a place of natural beauty and just sit there doing nothing. Doing nothing isn't easy; it takes discipline to sit quietly.

Learn about biofeedback as a way to discipline your mind. Discipline is important and improves with repetition.

Practice yoga postures, breathing exercises, and meditation. Your mind can't be tense if your body is relaxed. The mind will follow the body.

Regular exercise burns off aggressive energy and soothes the mind by producing calming endorphins. Only do exercises that you enjoy or else you'll find excuses not to exercise. Take a long walk and slow your breathing down .

Take warm baths, get a massage—anything that makes you feel good. Pamper yourself.

Do an arts-and-crafts project that takes your mind off your problems and focuses your thoughts on creating something you can take pride in.

Break up your unpleasnt routines. Take a short trip somewhere and get away from it all. Enjoy planning your trips because planning and looking forward to a trip are half the fun.

If you're having a really bad day, sit in your car with the windows rolled up and yell till you feel relieved.

Find sensible diversions to give your mind a break. To constantly dwell on your problems is depressing and unhealthy. You need diversions or you'll overdose on reality. It's OK to use diversions to avoid problems for a while. You can face the problems later when you're better able to deal with them.

Temporary denial isn't bad. However, only use diversions as a temporary way to gain relief and not as a permanent way to avoid thinking about things that you actually should think about. But, avoid escaping into the obvious diversions of overeating, alcohol, drugs, or maxing out your credit cards. Avoid bizarre and dangerous diversions like thrill seeking and extreme sports.

Summary:

There is no magic pill, no silver bullet, no special words of wisdom that instantaneously clears away stress. In real life, improvement comes slowly as the mind allows itself to face the problem in manageable bites. Attempts to swallow the whole problem at once will choke you.

Every problem is not solvable with a perfect result. Sometimes there isn't a good solution. It is then up to you to learn how to live with the problem by minimizing its stressful effects. Though there are some things we cannot change, we can change how we react to them. It's okay to be depressed at times. You're human. That's what human beings feel. It's nature's way of unloading.

Overcoming the negative effects of stress takes time. It didn't build up overnight, it won't leave overnight. The mind is a tremendously adaptable organ that can adjust to almost any stressful situation if given enough time and effort. Sometimes you may not feel you're making progress, but in moments of insight, you'll realize things seem a little better today than yesterday. You'll feel it happening, one small breakthrough at a time. Something that made you feel stressed last week, doesn't seem as important today. You'll feel stress tapering down, one tiny bit at a time.

Take care of yourself before you reach the critical stage. Do the common-sense things that keep stress under control. It's not an impossible goal. With the right frame of mind, things can work out and be better than you ever imagined. Once you've regained control of your life, you can slowly start to return to normal living while continuing to use the stress control aids that got you back on track. Be pragmatic. Do what works for you. If something seems logical but doesn't work for you, drop it. Don't get too analytical, just follow whatever you've learned is useful for you. Trust your instincts.

You will always have some stress. It's a part of our daily lives because our lives are constantly changing. Nothing is permanent. We have to stay aware of our stress level and make adjustments when necessary. Life is a neverending process of adapting to change.

Be gentle with yourself. Treat yourself as well as you treat others. You're important too. Try not to be all-perfect, all-knowing. Keep expectations of yourself realistic. Constantly remind yourself of your accomplishments. Pat yourself on the back once in a while. Find ways to reward yourself and don't depend on praise from others. Develop inner satisfaction and inner appreciation for the good things you accomplish. With the proper attitude and the right mind-set, you can endure and rediscover the joy of living.

Chapter 26

The Ingredients of A Good Nurse

"The making of a good nurse is like making
'jerk,' Jamaica's national food dish."
Florette Cramer, RN

The next morning, I mentioned the seminars on stress to Mrs. Cramer, "I learned a lot about stress I never knew. How about you? Have you ever felt stressed out and wanted to quit nursing?"

Cramer shrugged her shoulders and answered, "No, leaving nursing never occurred to me."

I was amazed that in all her years of nursing, under the most difficult circumstances, she had never once felt like quitting. I wanted to know more about her way of dealing with the pressures of nursing.

"Mrs. Cramer, how do you explain why many nurses burn out and you never even considered it?"

She answered crisply, "I enjoy working with patients and take pride in helping them get better and become more independent."

"What if they don't get better—or die?" I asked.

Her answer was clear, "There are no untimely deaths. Death comes when it is supposed to. It's a natural occurrence that I have no control over. A good nurse does her best and leaves the rest to God."

I said, "That makes sense. So what do you think makes a good nurse?"

She smiled broadly and said, "The making of a good nurse is like making Jamaica's national dish called 'jerk.' It takes many forms and there are many ways to make it, with no exact recipe. It's a way of taking a good basic main dish and adding a broad range of spices and special touches until you have a wonderful blend of ingredients. You sprinkle in a dash of cinnamon and sugar for extra sweetness. Then you slowly cook the mixture to allow time for all the good things to come together. If properly done, each result will be a unique creation. Since there is no exact recipe, there's always room for improvement. It's an ongoing effort to discover the potential of the mixture. It's more than a process, it's a way of life."

Cramer's quaint analogy painted a charming picture of the making of a good nurse.

Mrs. Cramer herself was a fine nurse and a good friend, but she always kept an unspoken distance between us. She never called me by my first name, therefore I never dared call her Florette—and certainly not Flo.

I mentioned it to her, "Mrs. Cramer, you've never called me John. In fact, you call all patients by their last names and they all call you Mrs. Cramer."

She replied, "It's more professional."

I asked, "What do you mean?"

"It's my way of showing respect for patients and them for me. You notice that doctors are never addressed by their first names. Addressing a patient as Mr. or Mrs. keeps the nurse-patient relationship in place. With disoriented patients, it keeps them grounded and aware of where they are. I don't want patients to forget that I am first and foremost their nurse."

Cramer saw I was interested so she explained further, "Nurses in pediatrics, geriatrics, and hospice can be less formal, but other nurses have to know the limits of familiarity. If a nurse becomes too casual, some patients won't show her the proper respect. It's no different than relationships outside the hospital, there are certain boundaries that shouldn't be crossed. That doesn't mean a nurse should be unfriendly, it just means she should behave in a professional manner."

I asked her if she followed any special guidelines.

She answered, "There isn't a step-by-step training method that lays it all out like placing footprints on the floor to learn how to dance. I just use common sense and learn from my mistakes. Nursing is a constant challenge and keeps you on your toes. That's what makes it fun."

Whatever Cramer was doing, it worked.

Having observed Cramer for almost two years, I had my own ideas of what made her such an excellent nurse. It started with her being a strong-minded woman with courage to follow her beliefs. She knew who she was and didn't depend on other people's opinions. Cramer wasn't trying to please everyone so they would like her. She wanted respect—not adulation. When she believed she was right, she followed through—no matter what. She was pragmatic and knew what worked and what didn't. The great nurses intuitively seemed to know what to do. Her methods didn't come out of textbooks, but I wished someone could capture them in writing so others might follow.

She once told me, "Nurses have to trust their instincts. They need to have the courage to do what they believe is right and stop second-guessing themselves."

Cramer told me she also trusted her instincts in raising her children. She had complete confidence in her child-raising methods and did what she thought was right, with no concern of being thought of as "too strict" or "old fashioned."

She said she provided her children with a structured environment with clear rules. One of her favorite expressions was, "You have to set limits." There was no wavering after a decision was made. Her children had to do what she expected of them. Despite her strictness, they sensed she was doing what was best for them.

Cramer explained how she raised her children with tough love. She firmly believed that discipline was necessary in raising children and didn't hesitate to punish them when they deserved it. When she took a switch to their backsides, she made them go and pick out the branch themselves—and it better not be too thin.

In Jamaica, when her son Gary stayed out late one night, she said she locked the door and he had to sleep outside till morning.

I said, "Some people would say that was child abuse."

"Rubbish, it's child abuse when you don't set limits. Let me tell you about the time when Gary wasn't at school when I went to pick him up."

She slipped into her Jamaican accent so I knew she wanted to make a point.

"One day Gary not dere when I come by to pick im up. He be messin roun and comin late I espect. I don wait, not me. Him not dere, I not dere. Im walk home lotsa mile. I nebba ask im how he comin home. When he get dere, im say I a wicked woman. But, I tell you, he nebba late agin. No mon, im always right on time."

I asked her how many children she had.

She slipped back into proper English and replied, "I have two. That's all I wanted."

I asked, "How many children did your husband want?"

She answered with a smile, "I never asked him." That was typical Cramer, always in charge.

Both of her children turned out well. Her daughter Althea was married with three children. She had a degree in social work and worked as a legal secretary. Her son Gary also had a family. He had a degree in business administration and a masters degree in law and was in private practice. They were all extremely close. She ended with, "It's all in the training."

Cramer was strict in training her patients too. She ran the ward with the same discipline and firm guidance, but behind the tough façade was a caring, compassionate nurse.

On the intermediate care ward, Cramer tended to patients with some of the worst diseases known to man. There were victims of cancer, strokes, diabetic complications, multiple sclerosis, Lou Gehrig's disease, and conditions with no medically known treatments, like mine. Cramer gave total patient care without regard to the effort involved.

As hard as she worked on the ward, she was able to flip that on-off switch in her mind when she was not on duty. Cramer had learned how to mentally separate the two different worlds. While on the ward, she could do the nastiest jobs without a second thought. She could remove impacted feces from a patient's rectum with a gloved finger, she could scrape off necrotic flesh from a cancerous foot, and do any unpleasant job on the ward without hesitation. However, once she left the ward, she flipped the switch and her mind was in a different place. In the hospital cafeteria, she sat away from patients with urine bags, IVs, and other reminders of the ward. At home too, she was able to tune out everything that happened on the ward that day. It was a mental discipline she developed over time.

Regarding her strict, no-nonsense way of nursing, I said, "You realize how rough you've been on me, don't you?"

She looked at me with wide-eyed innocence and said, "Have I now?"

I just shook my head and said, "As if you didn't know."

She dropped her innocence act and said, "Patients have told me they didn't like my firmness at first, but they later thanked me when they realized I cared about them and helped them get better. If a nurse is in touch with her patients, she'll have realistic expectations and know how far to push them—like I've done with you. That's why I became your primary nurse. Working in depth with patients reveals things about them that can't be discovered in team nursing. It also reveals things about yourself and how you can improve your nursing skills."

While I was on her ward, Cramer won the prestigious Hands and Heart Award in recognition of her nursing achievements. Humbly, she never mentioned it or displayed the certificate in her office. She wrote an article on nursing difficult patients that was published in the most prestigious nursing journal. But, external rewards were not that important to her. Her nursing accomplishments gave her internal rewards—the best kind.

The following day, I was walking on my walker in the halls when I found myself outside the swinging doors of the intensive care ward. I paused for a moment and wondered what it would be like to go inside and visit my old nurses. With a shrug of my shoulders, I thought, "Why not?"

I pushed the swinging doors open with one hand while I maneuvered my walker into the ICU. None of the nurses I knew were on duty. I was sure most of them had moved on to less demanding wards. The headnurse came over and asked if she could help me. I explained I had been a patient in ICU two years earlier and I just dropped in to say hello to my former nurses. She smiled and said I could stay as long as I wanted.

I stood quietly for a while, observing the patients who were as sick and scared as I had been. I could identify with what they were going through since I had had the same experience. I understood what they must be feeling.

I wondered if nurses could empathize with them as much as I could. I believed nurses could identify with the patients at some level since pain, depression, and suffering were common experiences for everyone, but there would be a difference in the degree of understanding. Unless a nurse had had a comparable experience in the past herself, she wouldn't be able to fully grasp the patient's state of mind. Her perception of all the things going on in a patient interaction would be different then the patient's experience--and also be different from another nurse's perceptions in the same situation.

I decided it wasn't possible for any two people to experience a situation in exactly the same way because perceptions were determined by the unique elements in each person's mind. Reality was distorted by the need to see what we wanted to see and believe what we wanted to believe, based on the need to fit things into our existing mental framework. Writer, Anais Nin said, "We don't see things as they are, we see them as *we* are."

It was probably good that a nurse wasn't able to completely relate to a patients' suffering or she would pay a terribly high emotional price. She might cross that invisibly fine line between being objectively empathic and being emotionally sympathetic wherein she felt what the patient felt.

My visit to ICU was complete and it was time to leave. I said goodbye to the headnurse and headed for ward 2-East. When I got back to my room, I found Dr. Strak waiting to say goodbye to me. His training at the hospital was done. We parted amiably.

During the course of our past discussions, I had gotten to see the person behind the psychologist's mask. Strak wasn't an unlikeable guy, but he wasn't someone I wanted to sit down and have a beer with either.

Through our conversations, he had revealed a side of himself that was rather antisocial—a trait of many psycho-therapists. I had once read that two out of three psychologists had problems with clinical depression themselves. This well-kept secret was the paradox of the mental health field. C'est la vie.

Fortunately, I had met some excellent psychotherapists. I believed good therapists were born, not made. The good therapists had an innate talent for understanding people that had very little to do with their academic training. You can't teach someone how to be perceptive, insightful, and compassionate. You either are or you aren't.

My counselor, Maryann, had that natural gift. There was no psycho-babble and no labeling in her counseling. She used simple, sensible, no-nonsense terms. As she listened to patients express their problems, she remained non-judgmental. Her ego stayed out of the therapeutic process.

She not only dealt with the everyday stresses of nurses and patients, she also dealt with their more troubling issues—though she did not get involved with mental illnesses caused by genetic factors or severe traumatic events that were beyond the scope of her pragmatic, non abstract methods of therapy.

In order to uncover broader issues for analysis, it was necessary for her to know the person's inner wants and needs. They were what motivated them. She told me, "If I know what your wants and needs are and how you satisfy them, I'll know who you are. They define you."

She then proceeded to explain her way of helping others.

"Basic needs are common to us all. They are in our DNA and we can't change them--though we can change our way of dealing with them and satisfying them. Obviously, we all have the inborn needs for survival, safety, avoidance of pain, and sex, but we also have inborn needs for love, belonging, self-importance, security, freedom, and independence.

"Wants are different; they are personal. We create them because we believe attaining them will make us happy. Many wants are foolish and unattainable, like wanting a perfect job with no pressures, wanting to keep our youthful looks, wanting to be loved by everyone. Tangibly, we want to own nice things, the more expensive, the better. Inwardly, we want structure in our lives, we want answers to the meaning of our lives, we want to stop the negative thoughts that disrupt our peace of mind. There are many other wants we aren't even aware of. We try to satisfy many of our wants in a hit-and-miss, disorganized way that becomes part of our troubled lifestyle.

"I believe that life is a journey of self-discovery. By discovering our motivations and our choices of behaviors to satisfy them, we get to understand who we are."

Through our many discussions, I got to know the methods Maryann used and the reasons behind them. I remembered her saying that in order to help patients, she first had to uncover and reveal their wants and needs. She said uncovering a person's inner wants and needs was done by examining ongoing behaviors. Wants and needs had to be identified, clarified, and held up to the light—hoping for an "Aha" moment. Negative emotions such as feelings of insecurity, inferiority, poor social relationships, dependency, and so on, were signals that some behaviors were dysfunctional and had to be examined and corrected. Once the source of a dysfunctional behavior was identified, she helped the patient put it in perspective, uncover the triggers that set it off, change how they chose to think about it, and understand it till it was neutralized and lost its power.

She understood the mind could not deal with larger problems all at once and it was best to face them in bite-size pieces. Getting to the source of a problem was like peeling an onion, one layer at a time. Wants had to be realistically attainable, socially acceptable, and contribute to self-growth.

Maryann offered a wealth of practical, proven, pragmatic ideas for patients to use in self-discovery. If patients became confused, she delicately guided them through the self-discovery process, encouraging them to, "Take all the time you need." Her expectations were realistic and her accepting attitude allowed patients to "just be who you are."

Maryann did not look for deep, dark secrets in the subconscious that only served to confuse the patient and made them feel a victim of uncontrollable forces. Rather than treating problems as a form of mental illness that required highly abstract methods whose history of effectiveness was questionable, she focused on the here and now, on current behaviors and attitudes. She only examined the past to show a person the wrong choices they had made—and also show them the right choices they had made that brought them to where they were today. If a chosen behavior did not move patients in the direction of their goal, it was replaced by a new, carefully thoughtout behavior.

Self-discovery required a plan of action for the patient. Maryann helped the patient create a workable plan, but it had to be the patient's plan, not hers. The patient was likely to need some suggestions from her, but the basic plan itself had to come from the patient. The foundation of a workable plan was the patients' belief in their ability to make changes, doing things that were under their control, and a commitment to carry it out. It was important for the patient to feel that he was in control of his own life and had the ability to make better choices. Once a plan was established, it was put in motion. It was important that the initial steps were small enough that the patient was certain to succeed in order to build confidence. For those things not under a patients control, like a basic need, there must be an acceptance and then a moving on.

When an immediate want or need was satisfied, a momentary feeling of "joy" was experienced. When a longterm feeling of well-being was experienced, a general state of "happiness" was felt. However, both joy and happiness were transitory; they came and went from time to time. New hopes and dreams became the new wants a patient believed would bring satisfaction, growth, and happiness.

Monitoring progress, or lack of progress, kept the patient on track. Wants and needs changed as the patient moved along the self-discovery path, so there was a need to make corrections along the way and adapt to life's everchanging flow. As life's conditions changed, so did the sense of self. No one was the same person today that he was yesterday. There was ongoing growth, regression, and regrowth, ad infinitum.

Maryann had been through the process of self-discovery in her own life and knew how to help others do the same. During the patient's journey toward self-discovery, she provided the human things every patient needed: thoughtful listening, caring attitude, and reassurance. Those were qualities I looked for in a therapist. I hoped everyone who sought psychological counseling would avoid the Dr. Strak type psychotherapists and instead looked for someone like Maryann, someone who didn't try to overwhelm them with psycho-babble and rigid, abstract theories, someone who helped them find their own way through the psychological mazes of life, and whenever they got lost, would take them by the hand and guide them onto the next rewarding pathway toward self-discovery.

Maryann recognized that self-discovery was never completed because the self was a dynamic force that continued to evolve and grow. However, the search lead patients to greater and greater understanding and satisfaction with their lives as the journey continued. Self-discovery was a remarkably fulfilling journey that had no final destination....

Thinking about how valuable she and my other nurses had been to my progress, I turned my thoughts toward writing an outline for the speech I'd be giving in three weeks at the student nurses' graduation. The writing went well. In an hour, I had roughed out a nice first draft. During the next two weeks, I rehearsed my speech, shaping and improving it until it finally felt right.

On the evening of gaduation ceremony, Cramer helped me get dressed. She had never tied a man's tie before, so I had to talk her through the steps. She helped me put on my sportcoat and folded the handkerchief in the jacket pocket. I was all set to go.

Cramer said she had some things to take care of that evening and was sorry she couldn't be at the ceremony.

At seven o'clock that evening, Meredith picked me up and drove us to the auditorium. As I sat in my wheelchair near the lectern waiting for my introduction, I looked out at the audience. There were parents, friends, and relatives of the nurses-to-be. I scanned the audience—and there in the rear row was Cramer....

When I was introduced, I felt calm and composed as I stood up from my wheelchair and steadied myself on the lectern. I had my speech thoroughly memorized so I was able to focus on my audience. My fifteen minute speech went exactly the way I planned. I spoke from my heart and told the graduates they had chosen the most noble profession in the world. I made them aware of how valuable nurses were and how nursing care had made the difference between my recovery and a bedridden life in a nursing home. I reminded them that the work they had chosen was often difficult and unappreciated, but it was the most rewarding thing they would ever do. One future day, when they looked back on their careers, they would be proud of themselves for the sacrifices they had made and the countless number of people they had helped. No profession offered more satisfaction. Most of all, I wanted to thank them for dedicating themselves to helping others. I ended with Albert Schweitzer's quote, "I do know this, you will always have happiness if you seek and find how to serve others."

When I finished, I received a hearty applause. The rest of the ceremony was thrilling. I enjoyed every minute as I watched each graduate receive his or her diploma. I knew many of them and I wished I could have personally congratulated each one on his or her achievement. The proud expressions on their faces said it all. These fine young women and men were beginning a new way of life that would constantly challenge their inner strength, demand their best, and reward them more than they could ever imagine....

Chapter 27

Attitude Is Everything

"As a man thinketh, so is he."
Thales, Greek philosopher

Today was really an upbeat day. My spirits were high because after two years and eight months in the hospital, I would be going home soon. I was planning for life outside the hospital and looking forward to my job interview later that afternoon. I was about to interview for a job that could change my whole life. I felt great. I was riding the wind.

I had planned today's activities carefully. I had everything scheduled in my mind. I'd get up at seven o'clock, wash, have breakfast, finish PT and be back in my room by eleven, practice my interview answers, change from pajamas to street clothes, eat a light lunch at noon, catch a taxi at one o'clock, and arrive at Northrop at 1:30 for my two o'clock appointment. I was on a mission.

After lunch, Cramer helped me dress and tie my tie. It felt tight around my neck and my sportcoat was starting to make me sweat. I was feeling nervous and took a few deep breaths to calm down before I left. I had Cramer phone for a taxi.

As I walked down the aisle on my walker, I saw the nurses watching me. Cramer and Redden were at the nurses' station smiling at me as I passed by. The other nurses on duty stopped their chores and came out of the patients' rooms to see me off. One of them said, "Good luck John" and started to clap. Soon they were all clapping and shouting, "Go get em John. " They were smiling, some were teary eyed—including me. This was their moment too. They had put in two years of hard work and sacrifice to get me this far. Cramer wished me luck with her typical, "Walk good mon."

I felt proud and inspired. I'd give this interview everything I had. This job would mean I could leave the hospital and support myself and my son. It was so important to my future that I had to put any thoughts of failing out of my mind.

The air felt warm and humid as I walked out the front door of the hospital. The taxi was waiting at the curb. I slid onto the front seat and the driver folded my walker and placed it on the rear seat.

The twenty minute drive on the freeway went fast as my eyes took in the sights. We arrived at the front gate of Northrop Corporation. The driver helped me out and set up my walker. I paid the fare and gave him a nice tip.

The security guard at the gate telephoned Tom to escort me into the building. In a few minutes, Tom arrived. He was his usual calm, smiling self. The last time he saw me, I was in pajamas, so he was surprised to see me all dressed up. We shook hands and exchanged greetings. It was a long walk from the gate to the manager's office, so by the time we reached the engineering department, I was sweating and a bit tired.

As soon as I walked into the large computer-filled room, some of my old buddies saw me and rushed over to greet me. I hadn't seen them in years. Though I was happy to see them, I felt embarrassed because I was on a walker and not the person they had known before. They didn't seem to mind.

Tom escorted me into Mr. Zane's office. He and I shook hands and he asked me to take a seat. Tom left.

I handed Mr. Zane a copy of my resume. Since my friends had told him all about me, he didn't have many questions. He put my resume aside and said he wouldn't need to read it. He asked me whether I thought I'd be able to work an eight hour day. I assured him it was no problem. I kept my hands out of sight as much as possible. I didn't want their limited use to negatively influence him. After ten minutes of pleasant conversation, he was satisfied that my health was good.

He said, "I think we'll give it a try, John. When can you start?" Just like that!

I told him I could start the first of the year, right after New Years. He wrote out a form for me to give to the personnel office. We shook hands and I left the office. On my way out, I waved goodbye to my buddies who were sitting at their computers. They all gave me "thumbs up. "

Tom escorted me to the personnel office. The young woman in personnel was extremely friendly. During our conversation, she told me she was taking care of her bedridden father who had had a paralyzing stroke. She and I instantly bonded.

After a few minutes of general conversation, she made me a salary offer I couldn't refuse. Upon our agreement of salary and start date, she filled out forms for me to sign. Our business was completed in an hour. The whole hiring process had been a very pleasant experience rather than the usually tense one.

She directed me to the medical clinic down the hall where I passed the basic physical exam with no problems. When the exam was complete, I had the nurse phone for a taxi and sat down to rest my tired legs. It had been a long day.

After a brief rest, I got up and went outside to wait for the taxi. It arrived in minutes.

On the way back to the hospital, I thought about everything that had happened. I was highly charged as I mentally reviewed the details over and over, talking out loud to myself. The driver probably thought I was nuts.

When I got back to the hospital, the afternoon shift nurses were on duty. Cramer had told Mrs. Agard where I was when she came on duty and Agard couldn't wait to find out what happened. When I told her I had gotten the job, she was as excited as I was. As she undid my tie and helped me off with my sportcoat, I filled her in on all the details.

I changed into my pajamas and got ready for dinner. I was famished. I had only eaten a light lunch and all the activity had given me an appetite. Dinner tasted especially good. After eating, I sat back in my wheelchair to think about the day's events.

I had mixed emotions. My thoughts bounced back and forth from elation to anxiety. I desperately wanted to get back to work and start a new life, but I couldn't help wondering whether I had reached too far, too fast? Had I forgotten everything I knew in the almost three years I'd been away? Could I really work eight hours a day without fatigue setting in? Could my hands and arms manage to manipulate the computer keys effectively? What did my old buddies really think of me as a handicapped person?

My head buzzed with thoughts and counter-thoughts. I muttered and mumbled to myself. My insecurities were being put to the supreme test. I swore out loud. I was trying to go from thirty-two months of hospitalization to a whole new life in one giant step. It wouldn't seem like such a giant step if my hands and legs were fully functional—but they weren't!

I wondered, "Why had I even tried? Was it a bridge too far? Why not just forget the whole thing and accept myself as a handicapped person doomed to live in a nursing home?"

But, every time my thoughts reached a low point, something inside me fought back. I still had an inner strength, a pride in who I was, in spite of my disability. Somehow I believed I could make it if I didn't allow myself to wallow in self-pity. The temptation to feel sorry for myself needed to be replaced with the courage to keep believing in myself. I held on to those positive thoughts till bedtime and as I fell asleep.

When Cramer came in the next morning, I was anxious to tell her I got the job, but I wanted to wait until she asked me. She came into the room, said "Good morning, Mr. Sweeta," and cared for me like she always did. She didn't mention the job at all. I thought my head would burst waiting for her to ask. Not a word. Didn't she give a damn?

As she left the room, she stopped in the doorway and said matter-of-factly, "A hear-so ya nail da job bra. Nice going, John." That was the first time in over two and a half years she ever called me by my first name! That was beyond special. After she left, I felt tears streaming down my cheeks.

I was so high that day, I couldn't stop talking about the job and going home. I must have used up all my positive energy as I described everything in detail to anyone who would listen. I should have been more restrained because, in the process, I had drained all my positive emotional energy. I knew better than to be so manic and disturb my emotional balance.

My mental high slowly subsided into a low as my lingering doubts of whether I could make it on the outside took over. I'd be leaving the hospital in two weeks, but I didn't want to reveal my fear of leaving. I couldn't tell anyone about my anxieties. Cramer, Agard, Rick, Maryann and all the others had given too much for me to let them down by showing how I felt. I wanted them all to feel proud of their accomplishment in getting me this far. It wouldn't be fair to show them I was filled with doubts and in some ways wished I wasn't leaving. I wanted everyone to believe they'd done a good job and that I was on my way to a wonderful life outside the hospital.

I decided to hide my true feelings and pretend everything was fine instead of revealing I'd rather stay in the hospital where I felt accepted. I couldn't share my real feelings with anyone. I felt alone.

I thought about the patients who weren't going home. Two patients on the ward whom I knew well had reached the limit of hospital care and were being sent to nursing homes. One had MS and his condition was deteriorating; the other had had a severe stroke and was permanently paralyzed on one side. Both men were permanently bedridden and would need total care.

Each of them had a wife and teenage children who obviously loved them, but the families were not willing to have them come home. The families realized their beloved husbands and fathers required a huge amount of care and it would be a fulltime, exhausting job to care for them. Both families chose to have the men sent to nursing homes. Very few wives had the fortitude of Mrs. Martin.

Some of the patients felt it was heartless for the families not to take them home and care for them. I didn't feel that way. Once a total-care patient myself, I knew the enormous amount of time and effort required to take care of a patient in their condition—even for trained nurses. If these men were taken home, the lives of their families would be negatively affected. The feeding, bathing, grooming, toileting, exercising, and medicating would totally interfere with any hopes the wives and children had for a normal life. Everyone's life would be ruined.

To my way of thinking, that was not the best alternative. In a VA nursing home, the men would receive the care of trained people. The environment would not be as loving as in their own homes, but that was the trade-off. The men would have to accept the conditions of a nursing home in exchange for allowing their families to lead normal lives. I would have done the same if it had been necessary. It was just another one of life's realities that some problems don't have perfect solutions.

During my long hospital stay, I had felt self-conscious when visitors asked me how long I'd been in the hospital. When I told them, "Over two years," they always looked amazed because two years in a hospital was such a long time. I felt embarrassed and compelled to add, "I'll be out soon. I'm doing much better. Maybe I'll be going home in a few months."

It surprised me how fast my time in the hospital had passed. In some ways, it seemed like an eternity, but in other ways, the time had flashed by. The first year in Intensive Care and the Rehab Ward seemed endless, but the last year and a half was a blur of activity. Why did time seem so long in some ways, but so short in other ways?

My memory of entering the emergency room many months ago was just as vivid to me as my memory of shaving that morning. Memories of my youth seemed like only yesterday. I still identified with the young man I had been, and not the man I now saw in the mirror.

Inside me somewhere, was still the young man I had been. Somewhere inside me was still the young soldier in the army, still the young man traveling through Europe, still the guy dating young girls. Why not? Those things were only a short time ago--weren't they?

Reflecting on my time in the hospital, led me to think about going home. When Thomas Wolfe wrote, "You can't go home again," he meant me. I was going home, but my life wouldn't be the same as it was. I would have to forget my past way of life. Like the old baseball player Satchel Paige said, "Don't look back cause somethin' might be gainin' on ya." I was going home and I had to look forward, not backward.

For one thing, I would have to drive a car to get to work. My right leg was fairly strong, but my left leg was weak. The motor nerves in my feet had not regenerated, so I had no movement below my ankles. With those limitations, I didn't know whether I could drive a regular car with foot pedals or if I needed hand controls? My hands were not fully functioning either. How would I grip the wheel to steer?

Rick told me there were ways to drive with my limitations and he arranged an appointment with the hospital's driver-training department.

When I talked with the young woman who was the driving instructor, she thoroughly checked my physical abilities by testing me on special equipment. To my surprise, she said I had excellent potential to learn how to drive, even with my disabilities.

The next day, she escorted me to the parking lot where she had me sit in the driver's seat of an Olds Cutlass with special modifications and dual controls. My hands were able to grip the steering wheel well enough to turn it. The only modification she set up was a reversed foot pedal attachment that would allow me to use my stronger right leg for braking and my left leg for accelerating.

It felt wonderful to sit behind the wheel. I was actually going to drive! She started the engine and told me to pull the gearshift into the drive position. I did. Next, she asked me to gently push down on the accelerator with my left foot while keeping my right foot poised on the brake pedal. My thigh muscles were able to push my feet downward so that the lack of foot movement didn't matter. We began to move forward slowly. I was driving! After moving a few yards, she had me brake. We repeated the gas and brake pedal coordination until I was able to do it well.

We drove around the parking lot until I got the feel of driving with reversed pedals. On the following days, we progressed to driving on streets around the hospital and finally to driving on the freeway. I drove with no problems at all. After five lessons, my instructor pronounced me ready to get a license once I was discharged from the hospital. Another large hurdle had been cleared. It was a giant step toward functioning independently outside the hospital.

During the past years, I had yearned for the day when I'd be able to leave the hospital and rejoin the real world. The months of struggle seemed endless and the frustrations had been almost unbearable. Now that those worst days were behind me and I was going home, I wondered whether the old saying was true that, "Happiness is in the journey, not the destination"—or was that another one of those Far East sayings that sounded profound, but was really only a hollow phrase? Would I look back on my months of struggle in the hospital with greater fondness than my life after my discharge?

I remembered seeing successful people on television saying their greatest pleasure was during the challenging days before they succeeded—even though success seemed doubtful at the time. Once they had reached their goals, they said their achievements seemed anticlimactic and not as fulfilling as they had imagined. They looked back at their journey as the true time of joy.

Were they rationalizing? Were my challenging times with its hopes and dreams to get off the ventilator and to walk more fulfilling than when I could actually breathe on my own and use a walker?

I decided it was quite the opposite. Even though I might look back at my time of struggle as a time of hope and anticipation, I was consumed with fears and the troubling uncertainty of how it would all turn out. If during those dark days, I had known I would achieve important goals, I might have taken more joy in the journey—but I hadn't known.

My conclusion was that my greatest feelings of joy were in the afterglow of reflecting back on the victories I achieved. The struggle itself wasn't enjoyable, it was the good feeling I got when I reflected back on my persistence and courage to overcome obstacles during the struggle. The destination was definitely better than the journey. However, I wished I had taken more joy in each bit of progress during the journey. I wished I had savored the small successes and smelled the roses along the way.

I also wished I had shown more gratitude for all the small acts of kindness that were shown to me during my journey. I had expressed my gratitude for the larger acts of kindness, but not the smaller acts. I thanked Theresa for allowing me to remain in ICU until I was off the ventilator. I told Rosa I was grateful to her for finding me when the ventilator hose became disconnected. Each of those incidents probably saved my life. But, expressing gratitude shouldn't only be for extraordinary acts.

I wished I had shown more appreciation for the many smaller things that nurses did for me. I was the fortunate recipient of many smaller acts of kindness, but it had been easy for me to overlook them because I was usually thinking ahead and not living in the moment. I was so wrapped up in my own self, I seldom showed nurses the gratitude they deserved. Making me comfortable, bringing me food from home, handwashing my underwear, grooming me, hugging me, encouraging me when I felt down—those things mattered too. Each one of those small kindnesses contributed to my comfort and peace of mind.

Whenever I did show my gratitude and recognize smaller kindnesses for the gifts they were, I saw the humanity behind the giving. Expressing gratitude connected me with nurses at a level that was simple, yet intimate. The joy of everyday living was in the small, warm human interactions.

One person to whom I showed my gratitude for all he had done, was my friend Hugh. Today we were going to look for a car and an apartment. Hopefully, we'd be able to find a car and a place that suited my disabilities and readied me for life outside the hospital. Maybe we'd have time for a chilidog.

Hugh arrived soon after breakfast. We left immediately and in an hour arrived in Redondo Beach. We bought the local newspaper and found an ad for an Oldsmobile Cutlass that sounded promising. As luck would have it, the car was exactly like the one I had trained on at the hospital, except for the special accelerator extension that allowed me to switch my feet.

Hugh took it for a testdrive because I needed the reversed pedal footbar to drive. It checked out perfectly and we bought it immediately. We both felt fortunate we had found the right car so quickly. Hugh said he'd install the footbar before I was discharged.

It was lunchtime. Hugh asked me what I wanted to eat. I didn't hesitate an instant, "I want a chilidog!"

Hugh looked puzzled by my enthusiasm about a mere hotdog.

I explained, "Hugh, I've been dying for a chilidog for over two years. You have no idea how many patients have told me they craved a chilidog. Did you know the Red Cross asked soldiers returning from Vietnam what food they missed the most, and the majority answered a chilidog."

He seemed amused and headed for world-famous Pinks where they had the best.

In a short while, I was sitting at an outdoor table with two big fat hotdogs smothered in chili and covered with onions and shredded cheese. The smell was intoxicating. I carefully picked one up, trying not to spill one bit of chili.

I bit into heaven. The spicy chili, tangy onions, and creamy cheese flavors exploded on my taste buds. I concentrated on each flavor as I chewed each bite twice as long as normally. I didn't want to miss a thing. I wanted to savor every morsel. This was one time when reality lived up to expectation. The flavors were even more delicious than I had imagined. I wasn't disappointed one bit. Was this living at its best or what?

Hugh didn't try to make conversation. He just smiled as he watched me lovingly enjoy the two chilidogs, one slow bite at a time. When the last bite disappeared, I sat back with my eyes closed to enjoy the aftertastes.

After waiting a few minutes, Hugh interrupted my reverie, "All done, John?"

I sighed with a smile of satisfaction, "Yeah, all's well with the world."

It was time to roll. Next on our agenda was a place for me and Chris to live. We scoured the ads and found a few possibilities. First, we checked out a house for rent, but I couldn't manage the steps in front.

The next place we checked was an apartment building on the Esplanade. It was a beautiful, three-story building right on the beach. It had underground parking and an elevator. We both liked the apartment and the location—who wouldn't? I wrote a check for the first and last month's rent. We had accomplished both missions in only a few hours. Sometimes things went right.

On the drive back to the hospital, good old Hugh said he would move my furniture out of storage and he and Chris would get it all set up for my return.

Back at the hospital, I gave Hugh a warm handshake and a sincere "thanks" before he left. He was the best friend anyone could have.

Well, it was all coming together. In a few days I'd be leaving the hospital and starting a whole new life. The thought was both exciting and scary.

During one of our afternoon conversations, Cramer told me that my progress was the highlight of her long nursing career. Her compliment lifted my spirits because it gave meaning to what I had endured. My struggle hadn't been for nothing. It had rewarded a great nurse for her lifelong commitment to nursing.

But, her compliment also put an obligation on me. Because she had put so much time and hard work into my care, I felt I couldn't let her down. I had to be worthy of Cramer's efforts—as well as the efforts of others—and continue to succeed after discharge. I had to stay motivated so I wouldn't disappoint them. My success might also inspire them to help other patients in a similar condition.

During the past year, I was never quite sure whether I had been driven to make progress for myself or for those who helped me. Did Cramer know the psychological obligation to succed that her devotion placed on me when she became my primary nurse? I wouldn't put it past her.

My last few days in the hospital were passing quickly and it was Christmastime once again, my third and last in the hospital. Christmas was bittersweet. I was filled with both the joy of going home and the sadness of leaving the staff who had become dear to me. I was stepping out of one life and into another completely different. The adjustment would be enormous because the two ways of life were completely opposite.

On Christmas morning, I went to the special mass in the hospital chapel. The chapel was magnificently decorated for the holidays. There were fragrant bouquets of flowers everywhere. Patients, staff, and well-dressed visitors filled the pews. The atmosphere was solemn but filled with the holiday spirit. Father Hunkler gave a wonderful sermon of hope and thankfulness. It was the most wonderful mass I ever attended. I left the chapel emotionally high, filled with the spirit of Christmas.

Back on the ward, I went into the dayroom where we had a large tree and decorations galore. Visitors had brought bouquets of flowers and dishes filled with cookies and candy. Hugh and his wife Barbara brought presents. The nurses looked festive with orchid corsages someone had given them.

I played some carols on the piano and everyone sang along. It was a terrific time.

That afternoon, the Salvation Army band came on the ward and played Christmas songs while their volunteer helpers distributed gifts to every patient. After the band moved on, students from local highschools sang carols as they strolled the hallways. Christmas day was a continuous stream of music and happy wellwishers.

After an afternoon of warm interaction with patients, staff, and visitors, it was dinnertime. The menu was turkey, ham, and more side dishes than anyone could possibly eat. I stuffed myself.

Charlie and Suzie came by after dinner to pick up where the others had left off. I sat in the hall next to Charlie as he played his music. We reminisced about old times. Charlie was a great person for having devoted his whole life to bringing music, warm conversation, and hope to fellow veterans.

Besides playing music, Charlie had made three historical albums of patients, nurses, and doctors. He had taken Polaroid pictures of each person and had them write a short autobiography and whatever comments they wanted to include. If a patient wasn't well enough to write, Charlie wrote it per their dictation. Each page was done with his careful attention to detail.

As I thumbed through the albums, I saw photos and comments of past patients and staff. Many I recognized— some were now gone. It was a joy to see their photos and reflect back on those who had fought so courageously.The nurses and doctors had informally posed for their photos and wrote small, personal thoughts. The façade of job titles and hospital roles were all put aside. The pages were filled with people who were willing to bare a part of their inner selves. As I turned the pages and read their thoughts on their hospital experiences, I felt a closeness for the patients and staff that tragedy had brought together. Charlie's albums were a beautiful historical record that other hospitals would do well to emulate.

Why did Charlie devote his life in such a simple way? I believed the reasons were very basic. He liked helping people and it made him feel good doing it. Those were the best reasons in the world. In a way, he was a very fortunate man to have found such a rewarding way to devote his time and energy. He was a man with simple needs and found what most people search for all their lives and seldom find—a mission in life, a reason for living.

Later in the evening, as I quietly sat in my room thinking about what a wonderful Christmas it had been, a man walked into the room. He looked vaguely familiar.

"Hi John. Remember me? I'm Jim. I came to see you a couple of times. I wasn't very clear-headed at the time. Do you remember me?"

It hit me. This was Jim, the drunken guy who was crying and could barely walk and talk. Standing in front of me was a man who was clean shaven, well-dressed, and had a happy glow.

"I've been totally sober for two months now. I finally had hit bottom and now I'm going through the Twelve-Step Program. Virginia is my sponsor."

I was so impressed that my eyes teared up. Here was a man who was completely different than the ragged drunk I met many months ago. I couldn't believe the transition. Jim had reached a wonderful stage of recovery and had all the signs of a man who was on the road to recovery.

He sat down and we talked for over an hour. Jim's story was heartwarming. I listened with interest and total compassion. He described how he was living with a friend and had just landed a job at his former occupation as an accountant. He was a college graduate who had lost his way and fallen on hard times. But, now he was on his way back. After all he'd been through, I believed he "once was lost, but now was found." I didn't doubt his bright future for a minute.

Jim smiled warmly and wished me a "Merry Christmas" as he walked away to his new life.

I didn't want the day to end, but it was bedtime. It had been the best Christmas of my life, a day I would always remember. I closed my eyes and drifted off into a peaceful sleep....

I awoke to Cramer's lilting voice saying, "Good morning."

Christmas was over and I had a lot of things to do. I would be leaving soon and it was time to say my goodbyes to all those who had meant so much to my recovery. This was my last chance to thank them for their marvelous help.

After a full breakfast, I put on my dress shirt, pants, and sportcoat and left the ward on my walker. My first stop was the gym. I forgot that the staff had only seen me in pajamas for over two years, so when I walked in the door in regular clothes, their astonished expressions turned into broad smiles.

I went over to see Rick one last time to thank him for his many hours of lifting my heavy body, teaching me how to exercise, and giving me his moral support. We were both a bit teary-eyed as we shook hands goodbye. I promised to keep in touch—and I would.

His supervisor, Doug, was nearby. I thanked him for his advice on exercising after I had received so much conflicting advice from others. I also thanked Doug for counseling me and giving me a personal philosophy for living as a handicapped person.

One of the female therapists openly cried as I shook her hand and said goodbye. She had seen my progress from a completely helpless patient in pajamas to a man all dressed up and leaving the hospital to live a normal life in the outside world.

She was another example of hospital staff who seldom saw the results of their efforts. The physical therapists saw pitifully weak patients with all types of physical disabilities. Few severely disabled patients ever came back to thank them and let them see their labors were worth the countless hours of physical effort they put in. I felt like an Olympic athlete who was taking one last victory lap around the stadium.

The next stop on my list was OT and Judy. I wished I had been more appreciative of her efforts. During the time she had been my therapist, I had been struggling to improve and was often depressed and surly. I asked her to forgive my thoughtlessness. Of course she did.

I had a terrific group of visitors that afternoon. Rosa and three other former nurses came by to visit. Somehow they had heard I was leaving and came to say goodbye.

I was now a totally different person from the patient they had first known. I was sitting erect and breathing on my own, not lying down with tubes stuck in my throat, arms, and foot. I was dressed nicely and not in wrinkled pajamas. They saw tangible proof of the value of their nursing. My improvement validated their nursing skills and efforts. I saw in their eyes and heard in their voices, the tremendous pride they took in seeing a former patient doing so well after such a terrible beginning. Instead of seeing only sick and dying patients day after day, they saw someone who was going home to lead a normal life. We had a wonderful, heartfelt reunion and I thanked them for all their help.

After we had said our long goodbyes, I thought about how seldom nurses were rewarded by seeing former patients who were doing well. Patients who went home rarely returned to thank their nurses and show them their nursing efforts hadn't been in vain. Most nurses got very little positive feedback, few pats on the back, hardly any strokes for a job well done. Nurses were on a one-way street where their energies flowed out but replenishing energy from others seldom flowed back in. Whenever nurses did have a chance to see the fruits of their labor, it justified their decision to become nurses. For one shining moment it all seemed worthwhile. If patients knew how important it was to return and thank their former nurses, maybe there wouldn't be so many good nurses burning out from the lack of nourishment to their nursing souls.

My goodbyes had all been said. It was time to go....

Chapter 28

Going Home

"Oh, to be home again, home again, home again!"
James Thomas Fields (1817-1881)

The chief of the research department, Dr. Jamison, came to have a chat with me before I left. He wanted to inform me of the latest medical developments in paralysis research. Many new things were happening in the field.

"John, there is a lot of research going on now in the field of neuronal regeneration. It may be a little late to help you, but many others will benefit from it in the near future. I have to admit that at the present time, we still don't have any major breakthroughs, but many research studies look promising. These treatments will help not only Guillain Barré patients, but others with MS, Parkinsons, ALS, and spinal cord injuries.

"In the area of neurochemistry, we're working on a potassium channel-blocking agent that should increase nerve conduction. Researchers are trying to find the switch that turns on the body's own myelin production. That would be the ideal solution. Unfortunately, the body has a natural tendency to inhibit regeneration of spinal nerves and we need to find an antibody. We are trying intravenous gamma globulin, which is an antibody concentrated to assist in regenerating nerve fibers.

"Plasmapheresis is another method in use. A patient's blood is filtered through a machine to separate the liquid plasma and replace it with saline, albumin, or special donor plasma. It removes the anti-bodies that are attacking the nerves. However, so far, the results are questionable.

"Corticosteroids are used sometimes, but the results aren't conclusive either.

"Another exciting area of research is cell transplantation. One method is to transplant myelin-forming Schwann cells. Another transplantation method uses stem cells from fetal tissue, but there are ethical issues involved. However, we hope to get stem cells from cloning our own stem cells and eliminate the ethical considerations.

"The Human Genome Project has recently mapped our DNA and it should incredibly speed up research in gene therapy.

"Any of these future medical treatments won't be instant cures. In medicine we don't like to use the term 'cure.' What we hope they will do is help in regenerating nerve cells. With the proper nutrition and rehabilitation, they should improve muscle functioning. How far it will go, we won't know until we're in full swing.

"For minor peripheral neuropathy which afflicts about 20% of older Americans with numb, aching feet and hands, we have topical Capsaicin ointment available. We've found that Vitamin B12, fish oil, zinc, selenium, and magnesium also help to improve the condition.

"So you see, John, there are a lot of things going on in the field. Who knows, maybe one of them will help you in some way."

Dr. Jamison smiled, shook my hand goodbye, and wished me luck.

After he left, I remembered my meeting with the federal committee that had visited the hospital last month to interview patients to see about improving the system. In the meeting, I had told them about the need to redesign the dangerously faulty ventilator hose coupling that almost killed me. I also had expressed my belief that patients should be included as partners in their own treatments. I hoped the committee would act on these suggestions and put them into practice.

As the hours passed while waiting for Hugh to arrive later, I reflected on my time in the hospital.

The hospital was a place all its own. The outside world was shut out. Everything I had needed was in that one building. It had been my life. Now, after almost three, long years, it was finally time to leave. Hugh would arrive soon to drive me home.

Mrs. Agard was busy packing my belongings into a cardboard box while I sat in my wheelchair looking out the window. The weather outside was a crisp, cool December evening.

The ward was peacefully quiet as Mrs. Agard finished packing my few possessions. I looked around my small room and thought about my present condition. My legs had not fully recovered, so I still needed a walker to get around. I could move my fingers, but the muscles in my forearms had atrophied from disuse so I couldn't fully close my hands to grip things, though I was still able to use my hands to do the normal things I needed to do.

I thought about Whittier's poetic words, "For of all the sad words of tongue or pen, the saddest are these, 'It might have been.' "

What might have been if I had received range-of-motion for my hands daily from the day I was admitted? If I had, contractures might never have developed in the joints and my hands would now be fully functioning. The contractures might also have been prevented if I had had an occupational therapist with very strong hands and the motivation to deep massage my hands for hundreds of repetitions every day. That was a lot to expect.

What if the ventilator weaning had been fully explained to me during the process? If that had been done, many of my deep fears would have been alleviated. The secretive way it was done was incredibly more upsetting than if each step had been explained as it occurred and I had been made a partner in the process. The staff should have realized I was mentally alert and capable of understanding.

What if my trach tube had been removed as soon as I was off the ventilator? If that had been done, I might have avoided many months of suctioning due to the foreign object in my throat. All those fears of suffocating on the rehab ward need never have happened.

What if Rick had been assigned to me for four hours every day to help me walk? Knowing someone was there who was strong enough to catch me if my knees buckled would have allowed me to push myself to my limit and not worry about hurting myself if I fell. In time, I might have developed my leg muscles and never needed a walker again. Unfortunately, the hospital couldn't give me that much of Rick's time.

On the other hand, I had a lot to be thankful for. I was thankful for many "what ifs" that went in my favor.

What if I had fallen asleep that night at Charlene's house or if she hadn't heard me calling her? What if her car hadn't started? I never would have made it to the hospital in time.

What if my heart hadn't been strong enough to sustain me through six months on the ventilator and the traumas afterward?

What if the Code Blue Team hadn't been able to revive me in ICU or if I had sustained brain damage before they did?

What if the nursing aide in rehab hadn't immediately answered my call-button when I was suffocating?

What if my nerve regeneration had stopped much earlier than it did? I might have ended up a permanent bed patient on a ventilator for the rest of my life.

What if Cramer hadn't taken me over and delivered primary nursing care? I might have remained in the condition I was in when she first took over.

What if I had never regained my swallowing muscles and had to be fed through an NG tube for life?

What if my vocal chords had been damaged during the tracheotomy or through necrosis and I was permanently voiceless?

What if I wasn't able to return to work and establish a normal way of life?

Yes, I had many more reasons to be grateful than regretful.

Sitting there in silence, staring out the window, my mind reflected back on all the tragedies and triumphs I had experienced in the hospital. Mental images of the past flashed in front of my mind like a motion picture. The reflections brought back memories of my difficult struggle to survive on the ventilator, the bitter conflicts with some staff members for trying to manage my own treatments, my depression from my slow progress, and my terrible fear of where it all might end.

I was not a perfect patient—few people are. I complained when I felt I wasn't getting the nursing care I needed. I got angry when frustrations overwhelmed me. Surviving a life threatening illness over such a long period of time was difficult for both me and the hospital staff.

However, mixed in with those unpleasant memories were memories of the good times. There were many. I smiled as I remembered all the wonderful friends I had made, the feeling of accomplishment I experienced at each stage of my physical progress, and the nurses and doctors who fought along with me and refused to let me fail. It had been a rollercoaster ride of extreme highs and lows. In the end, it all worked out.

I'd dearly miss Mrs. Agard, the grand old lady of nursing. She had two children but always wanted ten because she said, "It would have been wonderful to have had a home full of laughter." Her only son had died an early death. Her life had been one of tragedy and hardship, yet she always found time to help others, both as a nurse and as a patron to dozens of charities.

She told me about all the requests she got for donations. At last count, she was regularly sending contributions to twenty-two charities. She gave because she didn't know how *not* to give. She lived a life of endless self-sacrifice and gave all she had to give. She lived for others and had devoted her life to nursing. She was what all nurses should aspire to become.

Desdemona Agard had been my surrogate mother. She was my kind, sweet friend who did all the little things mothers do. She cared for me as if I were her son by encouraging me when I needed a lift, handwashing my T-shirts, and bringing me fresh fruit and home-cooked food.

I wished I hadn't taken for granted many of the things she did for me and all the wise things she taught me about life. She had a depth of knowledge I didn't fully appreciate at the time. I loved Mona without realizing how much. Shakespeare had his Desdemona and I had mine. I vowed I would never lose touch with her after I left the hospital.

I would truly miss Florette Cramer. She had been my inspiration, my motivator, my driving force. Her unflinching determination combined with her vast nursing skills made the difference between my returning to a normal life and ending up as a permanently bedridden patient in a nursing home. She drove, goaded, coaxed, scolded, yelled, and inspired me to keep trying even when it seemed pointless. She was relentless and didn't know the meaning of quit. I was blessed to have been the recipient of all her years of nursing experience.

Today she left work early so she wouldn't have to see me leave. She knew she would have gotten all teary-eyed and revealed what an emotional softie she really was. Behind that stern exterior was a sensitive human being. She hated being called "tough" and told me, "If I trust you, you can lead me around with a thread."

I'd miss all those wise old Jamaican sayings she quoted when she wanted to make a point. I'd miss our countless talks about nursing, raising children, and life in general. Many times we strongly disagreed—but never with a mean spirit. There was a mutual respect and genuine caring for one another. We had formed a deep nurse-patient bond. I would miss all of that. I once again remembered she had told me, "Of the thousands of patients I have cared for, your recovery has been the highlight of my nursing career." I made a solemn vow to live up to her devotion.

I had a lot of unanswered questions about myself. Would I be all right without nurses to help me if I had a problem? Would I be accepted in a non-hospital environment where others aren't used to dealing with disabled people? Could I function on the job as a handicapped person using a walker? Would I be able to start a whole new life with a son to raise? I didn't know the answer to any of these important questions. It was impossible to foresee how it would all turn out, but I reminded myself of the words of Invictus, "I am the master of my fate, I am the captain of my soul."

My thoughts were interrupted when Hugh walked into the room. My watch showed a few minutes past six o'clock.

"Hi John. Are you all ready to go?" He was smiling and filled with excitement.

Good old Hugh. It had been a long journey for him too. He had helped me through it all, faithfully visiting me every week, encouraging me, supporting me. I never knew anyone could be that giving. Friends like Hugh were rare.

"Yes Hugh, it's finally time for me to leave."

I sat in my wheelchair while Hugh placed the cardboard box with my belongings on my lap. He folded my walker and arranged it next to me so I could hold on to it and the box. Ready to leave, I was filled with mixed emotions. I was happy and sad at the same time. Happy to be leaving this place of suffering and going back to a whole new life, but sad to be leaving all the nurses, doctors, and therapists who had helped me. This had been my life and home for almost three, long years. I'd miss the halls where I had spent so many hours building up my leg strength. I'd miss the gym where I had sweated and strained month after month, winning and losing. I'd miss the cafeteria, the hospital store, and the library. I'd miss the whole damn place and all the people in it.

As Hugh got behind my wheelchair, Mrs. Agard bent down and kissed me on the cheek. I reached up and hugged her tightly. Hugh said goodbye to her as he wheeled me out the door and down the main aisle for the last time. We passed by the open doors of the other patients' rooms. I glanced inside at those who were never going to leave the hospital or else be shuttled off to a nursing home. Not many patients on this ward made it back to a normal life. I was one of the lucky ones.

We arrived at the elevators, waited briefly till one arrived, and got in. Hugh pressed button number 1, and the doors slowly closed, shutting out Ward 2-East and all the people I had been so close to for so very long.

I humbly remembered those nurses who gave me their all. I sadly wondered, "Who is going to take the places of these wonderful nurses when they retire? Who is going to save and rebuild lives like they did? Nursing is a profession of the highest nobility. It takes a special kind of person to shepherd the helpless and show compassion, patience, and grace under the most difficult circumstances."

I sincerely hoped there would be a new generation of dedicated young women and men coming to take their places. The need was critical.

Home...I was finally going home. A good job, an apartment on the beach, and a new life were waiting for me. It seemed ideal, yet I knew the adjustment would not be easy. Nothing worth having ever came easy. But, I hadn't come this far only to fail now.

I believed deep down in my heart that better days were ahead. I was going to make it work—Cramer would not accept anything less. I could hear her voice telling me, "Walk good, mon!"

www.ingramcontent.com/pod-product-compliance
Lightning Source LLC
Chambersburg PA
CBHW051449170526
45166CB00001B/170